**DO NOT REMOVE
CARDS FROM POCKET**

**ALLEN COUNTY PUBLIC LIBRARY**

**FORT WAYNE, INDIANA 46802**

You may return this book to any agency, branch,
or bookmobile of the Allen County Public Library.

# HEAVY DRINKING

# Heavy Drinking

## The Myth of Alcoholism as a Disease

Herbert Fingarette

University of California Press
Berkeley / Los Angeles / London

University of California Press
Berkeley and Los Angeles, California
University of California Press, Ltd.
London, England
© 1988 by
The Regents of the University of California
Printed in the United States of America
1  2  3  4  5  6  7  8  9

Library of Congress Cataloging-in-Publication Data

Fingarette, Herbert.
  Heavy drinking.

  Bibliography: p.
  Includes index.
  1. Alcoholism—United States.  2. Alcoholism—
United States—Prevention.  I. Title.
HV5292.F56  1988      362.2'928      87-26692
ISBN 0-520-06290-6 (alk. paper)

To my beloved grandson ANDREW, now
seven years old, whose charm and wit
provided a joyful counterpoint to the
labors of writing this book.

# CONTENTS

# ACKNOWLEDGMENTS

A good part of the work on this book was done while I was a fellow at the Center for Advanced Study in the Behavioral Sciences at Stanford, California. I am pleased to express my appreciation to the staff for the remarkable cordiality of their hospitality, and my gratefulness to the Center for providing me with important financial support and the opportunity to spend a year of undistracted work in the Center's attractive physical setting. To this I add my sincere thanks to the Mellon Foundation for its generous financial support during that same year.

I wish also to acknowledge the moral and financial support I received from the national liberal arts scholarship society Phi Beta Kappa, which designated me Romanell–Phi Beta Kappa Professor in Philosophy for 1983–1984. That honor provided the occasion for me to deliver three inaugural lectures, in one of which I first set out in brief form the main lines of thought elaborated in this book.

My daughter, Ann Fingarette Hasse, who has also at times been my co-author, read a late-stage version of the manuscript for this book. She provided me with insightful, incisive, and constructive editorial advice.

Amy Einsohn has been an incomparable editor. Her work on every aspect of the manuscript has been unstinting and her editorial insight and skills superb. No author could have hoped for more.

My wife, Leslie, has lived through this book with me, as with all my books. In daily and wonderful collaboration, she is not only my very competent secretary but also a keen, tough editor, an unflappable critic who knows when to be patient— and when to be impatient. Fortune has been kind to me.

# What Science Now Knows, but the Public Doesn't

*Another* book on alcoholism? Why? Oddly enough, and despite the many books on the topic, there is an important untold story: Almost everything that the American public believes to be the scientific truth about alcoholism is false.

The facts are an open secret. That is, they are quite familiar to scientists and leading researchers in a variety of fields who read the major journals and books addressed to professionals. Indeed, the relevant scientific literature spans several decades of research that roundly contradicts popular beliefs and suggests an entirely new perspective on alcoholism and heavy drinking.

And yet the public—including many counselors and paraprofessionals working in treatment centers—remains in the dark, still holding, and encouraged to hold, beliefs that are forty years out of date.

The aim of this book is to bring the major findings of mainstream science—biology, medicine, psychology, and soci-

1

ology—to the attention of the general public. In order to do so, I devote Part One to a critique of the account that the general public still believes, the classic disease concept of alcoholism. There I explain how and why researchers have come to know that this traditional concept is inadequate and incorrect. In Part Two, I introduce the new scientific perspectives on alcoholic use and abuse and describe constructive approaches for researchers, public-policy makers, treatment program staff, and heavy drinkers who are seeking help.

A few remarks on the style and form of this book. I have tried to present an account that is reliable, responsible, and readable. To this end, I have kept the documentation of sources brief and omitted some of the intricate detail and qualifications that are necessary to the working scientist but not to the general reader. Complete entries for all works mentioned in the end-of-chapter notes are provided in the section Works Cited. Readers familiar with the field will, I trust, agree that the authorities I cite are among the most eminent experts and represent the spectrum of current views.

Of course, no one expert or experimental study is beyond criticism, and each finding that I cite could provoke a lengthy analysis of the finer points of scientific method and technique. But my arguments are derived from the overall preponderance of evidence, not from any one set of studies by any one school of researchers.

## The Great Myth:
## The Classic Disease Concept

What is the "classic disease concept of alcoholism"? First proposed in the late 1930s, it goes like this. Alcoholism is a specific disease to which some people are vulnerable. Those who are vulnerable develop the disease if they take up drinking. From apparently normal social drinking, they progress to drinking ever greater amounts, to private and secret drinking, to developing an increased tolerance to liquor, and to experiencing withdrawal distress if drinking is interrupted; they begin to have blackouts (morning-after amnesia) and they forget the previous day's drinking bout. Most crucially: those afflicted by the disease *inevitably* progress to uncontrolled drinking because the disease produces a distinctive disability—"loss of control," a loss of "the power of choice in the matter of drinking."[1] Then, as the saying goes: One drink, one drunk.

According to this disease concept, alcoholism progresses stage by stage in a regular, fairly standard course that does not respect a person's individual characteristics: "Background, environment, race, sex, social status—these make no appreciable difference when once the disease takes hold of the individual. For all intents and purposes he might just as well then be labelled with a number: he has become just another victim of the disease of alcoholism."[2] Inevitably, the alcoholic "hits bottom." From there, physical or emotional breakdown and premature death is the final step unless, with luck, or God's grace, or the help of Alcoholics Anonymous or some sort of treatment, the drinker manages a radical conversion to total abstention. Abstention is the only hope, because the disease is incurable. At best, an alcoholic learns to abstain from the fatal first drink that invariably triggers a new descent into drunken oblivion.

Few people (except those involved with alcoholics) can fully state this entire theory, and many people either do not believe every detail of the doctrine or hold some beliefs inconsistent with it. But versions of the classic disease concept remain a dominant theme in the public's thinking about alcohol abuse.[3]

And yet, *no* leading research authorities accept the classic disease concept. One researcher puts it quite baldly: "There is no adequate empirical substantiation for the basic tenets of the classic disease concept of alcoholism."[4] Another expert, whose views are more conservative, dismisses the classic disease concept of alcoholism as "old and biased," a model whose propositions are "invalid."[5]

Scientific evidence or no, many knowledgeable people are greatly disturbed by criticism of the disease concept. They argue that the labeling of alcoholism as a disease frees alcohol abusers from feeling guilty or ashamed of their drinking and thereby makes it easier for them to seek treatment. This has the ring of plausibility, and yet reports suggest that the disease concept does not always have this effect. Many heavy drinkers view the labels "diseased" and "alcoholic" as stigmatizing, and so they reject help under such terms.[6] Furthermore, the notion that this disease causes people to lose the ability to control their drinking may discourage a heavy drinker from trying to stop in the (false) belief that it's hopeless. Then, too, some drinkers will not seek help if they believe that lifelong abstinence is the only "remedy" for uncontrolled heavy drinking; the thought of never being able to have even an occasional social drink is too disheartening. Finally, proponents of arguments for retaining the disease concept as a useful tool take it for granted that getting the drinker into alcoholism treatment will make a big difference—an assumption that is not supported by the scientific evidence, as we shall see.

## The "Other" Heavy Drinkers

Perhaps most important, however, is the fact that the preceding debate misses a much larger issue. The classic disease concept of alcoholism is unquestionably a hindrance rather than a help in addressing the broad problems of heavy drinking in our society. This is because most individuals in the United States who drink heavily and who get into most of the troubles related to alcohol do not think of themselves as alcoholics and would not be diagnosed as alcoholics.[7] Not surprisingly, then, very few of these heavy drinkers receive any professional help.[8]

Who are these "other" heavy drinkers? They are people who drink a lot and acknowledge it, but insist, "I can handle it." They get into serious trouble, but they say, "Everyone has family troubles, or job, or money, or other troubles sometimes." They point to some particular difference between their own cases and the many possible "symptoms" of alcoholism: "I don't lose control; I know what I'm doing"; "I never drink as much as a fifth of liquor a day"; "I don't have blackouts"; "I'm carrying on at my job"; "I'm not always drunk."

The litany of excuses and denials is endless. These people deny the significance of their heavy drinking and life problems by showing, often quite correctly, that in one respect or another they do not fit the profile of symptoms of the so-called disease. In this way, the prevalence of the disease concept narrows the scope of inquiry, concern, and help.

For example, it is well known among specialists that there is no clear-cut objective line between "alcoholics" and "problem drinkers." The figures published about the number of alcoholics in the nation often represent the propaganda intent of the agency or institute issuing the data. (Government alcoholism agencies and treatment centers typically publicize the most frightening numbers in order to call attention to the issue.) Depending on the definitions and statistical techniques used, the estimated number of "alcoholics" in the U.S. can range from near zero to as many as 10 million or more.[9]

But another picture of drinking problems emerges if we turn from the misleading black-or-white issue of "alcoholics," and instead examine consumption and a wide range of alcohol-related problems in domestic, job, money, health, and police matters. At any given time approximately 20 percent of the U.S. population drinks enough to be, on a statistical basis, at substantial risk of having alcohol-related problems. That is a very high figure indeed—and it includes persons of all ages and a significant number of women, although the single largest at-risk group consists of young adult males. By far the greater number of these problem drinkers do *not* fit any of the traditional diagnoses as alcoholics.[10]

This is a crude measure, but a telling one, of the scale on which the focus of public attention and resources has been misdirected. After all, it is this large group that generates most of the alcohol-related problems in the nation. Although their individual problems may be fewer than those of diagnosed alcoholics, these heavy drinkers are so much more numerous that their aggregate problems are far greater.

Meanwhile, researchers who have worked on the problems of heavy drinkers have devised new conceptual approaches. First, it is now a truism in alcohol research that there are crucial psychological and social dimensions to problem drinking, that economics and politics, cultural norms, and cultural stereotypes play a significant role. Second, it is a truism that heavy drinkers do not constitute one homogeneous group suffering from one "disease." Heavy drinkers are a diverse lot, differing in individual motives and patterns of drinking, in life settings and ways of living. Thus rather than seeing one disease (alcoholism) with one cure (abstinence), researchers are looking at heavy drinking as a behavior that serves different functions and fulfills different needs for various individuals.

Because there are so many different patterns of chronic alcohol abuse, I use the phrase *heavy drinking* as the general label for all forms of excessive consumption, reserving the word *alcoholism* for reporting the work of researchers who use that term in their studies.

## Dependence, Compulsions, Addictions

From what I have said, you may already be wondering how the new approach to alcohol abuse bears on other forms of addiction or compulsive behavior. What about addictions to heroin, cigarettes, caffeine, cocaine, gambling? What about compulsive eating, or compulsive spending, or repeated sexual offenses?

The pattern of chronic heavy drinking seems at least somewhat analogous to these other patterns of behavior, all of which we tend to refer to as addictions, compulsions, or dependence. And some researchers are starting to conceive of all these forms of "excessive appetite" as variants on one theme, to be incorporated in a "unitary theory." [11] This idea is still somewhat speculative, however, and despite the important commonalities, the evidence also shows significant differences—behavioral as well as chemical—among the various so-called addictions.

Let me add that although I do believe that many of the basic ideas presented in this book apply equally well to other addictions, nothing in my discussion hangs on any such belief.

It may avoid confusion if I also add that this book is not primarily concerned with alcohol intoxication. [12] Obviously heavy drinkers are often intoxicated, but not everyone who gets intoxicated is a chronic heavy drinker. On the contrary, most people who get drunk on occasion are not chronic heavy drinkers. So, while the two topics can't be completely separated, this book focuses on chronic heavy drinkers and the difficulties of understanding and helping persistent long-term drinkers.

Notes

1. Mann, *Primer on Alcoholism* (1950), 8.
2. Mann (1950), 10.
3. *Alcohol: Use and Abuse in America* (1985); Caetano, "Public Opinions About Alcoholism and Its Treatment" (1987); Crawford, "Attitudes About Alcohol" (1987).
4. Marlatt, "The Controlled Drinking Controversy" (1983), 1107.
5. Kissin, "The Disease Concept of Alcoholism" (1983), 121.
6. Shaw et al., *Responding to Drinking Problems* (1978), 58–61.
7. On the self-perceptions of heavy drinkers, see M. Moore and Gerstein, *Alcohol and Public Policy* (1981), 44–45; Moser, *Prevention of Alcohol-Related Problems* (1980), 55–70. On the diagnosis of heavy drinkers, see Olson and Gerstein, *Alcohol in America* (1985), 22–23.
8. Saxe, Dougherty, and Esty, "The Effectiveness and Cost of Alcoholism Treatment" (1985), 488.
9. On the issue of measuring, see Room, "Measurement and Distribution of Drinking Patterns and Problems" (1977), 78–79; Cahalan, "Subcultural Differences in Drinking Behavior" (1978), 240; Schuckit, *Alcohol Patterns and Problems* (1985c), 32; Cahalan and Room, *Problem Drinking Among American Men* (1974), 29.
10. Statistics of this kind are highly variable, often depending on inferences as well as diverse definitions. See, for example, Saxe, Dougherty, and Esty (1985); Room (1977); Clark and Cahalan, "Changes in Problem Drinking Over a Four-Year Span" (1976).
11. Peele, *The Meaning of Addiction* (1985), is to my mind the best recent comprehensive statement about addiction. Peele draws on a variety of disciplines in his discussion of heavy drinking as a complex human dilemma rather than a unitary physical disease; see also Galizio and Maisto, *Determinants of Substance Abuse* (1985); Peele, *Visions of Addiction* (1987c); Orford, *Excessive Appetites* (1985). An interesting study of the psychosocial meaning of heroin addiction and recovery, which touches on themes in this book, is Biernacki, *Pathways from Heroin Addiction* (1986). See also Kaplan, *The Hardest Drug* (1983); Fingarette, "Addiction and Criminal Responsibility" (1975) and "Legal Aspects of Alcoholism and Other Addictions" (1981).

12. For a review of the effects of intoxication on behavior, see Room and Collins, *Alcohol and Disinhibition* (1981). On the legal aspects of intoxication, see Fingarette, "Excuse: Intoxication" (1984). A highly influential work that proposes a "social construction-ist" interpretation of intoxication, an approach compatible with that of this book, is MacAndrew and Edgerton, *Drunken Comportment* (1969); see also Chapter 3, note 13.

# PART 1

# The Classic Disease
# Concept of Alcoholism

# CHAPTER 1

# Where Did We Get the Idea That Alcoholism Is a Disease?

The proposition that alcoholism is a disease has not always been with us. Quite the contrary. Not until the middle of the twentieth century did the familiar classic disease concept emerge and take hold in our nation's public consciousness.

To appreciate how the classic disease concept came to the fore, we need first to place it in a historical context. As this retrospective will show, cultural values, rather than careful observation or scientific evidence, have been decisive right up to the present time in determining what Americans have taken to be the "facts" about alcohol use and abuse.

## Colonial America's Love Affair with Drink

The influential colonial preacher Increase Mather spoke of rum as "the good creature of God."[1] This attitude was in keeping with centuries of religious opinion on the matter. The early Church fathers, for example, accepted and even recommended the use of beer, wine, and distilled spirits. Mather's views were also representative of medical opinion of his era. Beer, cider, rum, gin, and brandy were believed to be nutritious and healthful for body and mind, good medicine for many ailments.[2]

In early America, indeed, some form of spirits—and in large quantity—was indispensable for collegial conviviality. When the Virginia Council of State convened, a brandy punch was always at hand, and councillors commonly were quite merry, if not drunk. During a dinner reception hosted by New York Governor De Witt Clinton for the ambassador from France, the 120 guests consumed 135 bottles of Madeira, 36 bottles of port, 60 bottles of beer, and 30 bowls of rum punch.[3]

There is no doubt that from early colonial days through the early nineteenth century, Americans drank far more alcohol than we do nowadays. Children were taught to drink at an early age, and men and women participated equally: "The general pattern for the eighteenth century was for men and women to drink alcohol every day, at all times throughout the day, and in large quantities on almost every special occasion."[4] Throughout the eighteenth century the average American downed 4 gallons of alcohol a year, compared to about 2.5 gallons a year per person in our era.[5] (We should note, of course, that per capita data conceal certain patterns. Today, for example, three-fourths of all the alcohol consumed in our country is drunk by about one-fifth of the population.)

I do not report these facts to defend or advocate such heavy drinking. The point is simply that early Americans had a very different attitude about alcohol use than we do. In those days, drinking was considered essential to daily sociability, although the quantities consumed may strike us as excessive.

Of course they got drunk at times. Occasional drunkenness was one of the natural consequences of social drinking. But Americans in the colonial period did not associate drunkenness with violence, crime, or even rowdiness. Antisocial drunkenness was ascribed to the frequenting of taverns favored by criminal or rowdy or shiftless people; it was the association with such people, not the alcohol, that seemed to cause problems. "Habitual drunkenness"—some of which we would today call "alcoholism"—was not viewed in terms of a "loss of control" or the onset of a disease. It was a matter of consuming too much of a good thing.[6] Some people eat more than is good for them, or they indulge excessively or inappropriately in sex, or they are spendthrifts. And some people habitually drink "more than is good for them," as we say.

I would not argue that our forebears were right and we are wrong. But from them we can learn that what appears at a given time to be self-evident or obvious about the significance of alcohol is often a reflection of cultural beliefs, the spirit of the times. Perhaps they were victims of their beliefs; but then so are we victims of ours.

## The Nineteenth-Century Reaction: "Disease" and Temperance

By the turn of the nineteenth century, America's social patterns and cultural beliefs were dramatically changing. A new mercantile work ethic began to replace the older pattern of agricultural subsistence labor and upper-class luxury and leisure. New mechanical inventions revolutionized the economy and seized the public imagination.

At this time, too, scientists were laying the foundations of modern astronomy, physics, and chemistry. Inspired by the mechanistic paradigms of the new physics and chemistry, physicians began to speculate in mechanical terms about human anatomy and physiology. Many believed, for example, that physical and mental ailments were the result of excess quantities of blood in the circulatory system, and bloodletting was a frequently prescribed cure. The concept of disease also became a touchstone in social thought. Moral and social ills were now perceived as pathologies of either the individual or the body politic.

Consistent with this new ideology, the proposition that habitual drunkenness was a disease rapidly gained currency. The principal propagator of this theory was Benjamin Rush, an enormously influential physician who also was among the first to argue that strange, extreme, or bizarre behavior and emotional states were caused by mental diseases.[7] Rush's work, of course, was pervaded by the erroneous notions of his times. His medical "explanations" concerning the causes, courses, and cures of various diseases today strike us as largely fanciful. And although Rush tried to substitute first-hand observation for theological doctrine, his writings contain very little of what we would call scientific evidence: no carefully controlled experiments, no statistical analysis of data.

But Rush's mechanistic assumptions about disease in general and the disease of alcoholism in particular spoke to the spirit of his time. The lack of scientific evidence and data were not remarkable, and there was a persuasiveness in the style of his arguments.

By the mid-nineteenth century, a complete turnabout in social attitudes toward alcohol was everywhere apparent. Beginning most dramatically between 1830 and 1850, per capita consumption dropped from a high of about 5 gallons a year to around 2.5 gallons, the level at which it has hovered ever since. One commentator, writing in the *North American Review*, summarized the new public mood when he argued that "[the] unrestricted manufacture and sale of ardent spirits is almost the sole cause of all the suffering, the poverty, and the crime to be found in the country."[8] "The good creature of God" had become "the demon rum."

The nascent temperance movement took the disease concept of alcoholism to its extreme, claiming that alcohol in *any* form would lead to habitual drunkenness in *anyone* who drank.[9] The only way to prevent the epidemic spread of the disease, temperance workers preached, was total prohibition. Like Rush, advocates of prohibition had no scientific or medical evidence for their position. Their appeal was an emotional one, based only on their faith in what seemed to them the self-evident truth about the poisonous power of alcohol.

## Prohibition and Repeal

In 1919 the temperance movement achieved its crowning success: the Eighteenth Amendment to the Constitution was ratified, prohibiting the production, sale, and transportation of intoxicating liquors for "beverage purposes." As we know, the ban proved impossible to implement and provoked an especially malevolent form of nationwide gangsterism. But Prohibition was apparently successful in reducing consumption, and alcohol-related health problems declined during the 1920s.

The repeal of Prohibition in 1933 was the outcome of complex political and social trends. What is particularly interesting to us is that this shift in public opinion about alcohol, like earlier changes in social attitudes, was a matter of sentiment and perception, not the result of any new scientific research. By the early 1930s the temperance notion of alcohol as a universally addicting substance had simply lost its grip on the American mind and political will.

Once the fervor died down, people recalled that Europe and the United States had a long cultural tradition of moderate social drinking and that the vast majority of social drinkers did not become habitual drunkards. Clearly, many people were capable of drinking alcohol without falling victim to it.

Despite the repeal of Prohibition, the temperance creed lingered on in some quarters. In 1935 the old doctrine was given new life by the founders of Alcoholics Anonymous (A.A.). Inspired by the teachings of a then popular religious sect, the Oxford movement, two reformed heavy drinkers, a stockbroker and a physician, proposed a less extreme version of the temperance thesis. Their new approach was in essence a mixture of pseudomedical, psychological, and religious ideas.[10]

According to the A.A. ideology, most people can drink socially without any problem. But some people have a unique biological vulnerability to alcohol and they develop a special kind of "allergy." For these at-risk drinkers (alcoholics), alcohol triggers an uncontrollable need for more alcohol. The only way that alcoholics can halt the progressive deterioration of alcoholism is by complete abstinence: "An alcoholic cannot be cured of his disease so that he can drink normally again."[11] If an alcoholic continues to drink he or she will, stage by stage, succumb to a disease that has only two outcomes, insanity or death.

A.A.'s teachings were derived from an amalgam of ideas that fit together only loosely. There are appeals to the alcoholic's willpower as well as an emphasis on his helplessness. In order to achieve abstinence, the alcoholic needs to acknowledge dependence on the help of others (specifically A.A.) and, ultimately, on a "Higher Power," but the nature of this power is left to the individual. Drinking is interpreted as a symptom of disease, and ritual public confession at A.A. meetings, the admission that one has an incurable vulnerability to alcohol, is a necessary part of the treatment.


## The Mantle of Science

For a decade or so, A.A. grew modestly. But, lacking scientific confirmation, it remained a relatively small sectarian

movement, occasionally receiving a boost in popular magazines. The great surge in the popularity of the A.A. disease
concept came when it received what seemed to be impeccable
scientific support. Two landmark articles by E. M. Jellinek,
published in 1946 and 1952, proposed a scientific understanding of alcoholism that seemed to confirm major elements of
the A.A. view.[12]

Jellinek, then a research professor in applied physiology at
Yale University, was a distinguished biostatistician and one of
the early leaders in the field of alcohol studies. In his first
paper he presented some eighty pages of elaborately detailed
description, statistics, and charts that depicted what he considered to be a typical or average alcoholic career. Jellinek cau-
tioned his readers about the limited nature of his data, and he
explicitly acknowledged differences among individual drinkers. But from the data's "suggestive" value, he proceeded to
develop a vividly detailed hypothesis.

Jellinek postulated a basic pattern of alcoholism that re-
markably paralleled the A.A. picture. The sequence of the
disease's key phases begins with apparently innocent social
drinking. Through an insidious process of increasing involvement with alcohol, the alcoholic loses control over his drinking and cannot stop once he has started. He then plunges into
an ineluctable and disastrous descent until he hits a "low
point." At that time, by an enormous effort and with the aid
of others, some alcoholics come to their senses and manage a
course of total abstinence.

It now seemed that A.A. teachings had been triumphantly
confirmed by scientific research. Jellinek's powerfully dramatic
description was buttressed by numerous statistical charts and
tables, by elaborate analyses of questionnaire data, and by all
the scholarly apparatus one would expect of a sophisticated
scientist. His descriptions of the archetypical alcoholic career
and even some of his charts were reproduced widely in popular periodicals, and a new national consensus about alcoholism began to coalesce.

In 1960 Jellinek published *The Disease Concept of Alcoholism*, a book that eventually became the canonical scientific text for the classical disease concept. By this time Jellinek had developed a more refined classification. He posited five main types of alcoholism, which he labeled with Greek letters. The classic American disease pattern now was baptized as *gamma alcoholism*.

Jellinek wavered as to whether loss of control always follows on the first drink. In the end he suggested that there were degrees of loss of control, and he proposed some working hypotheses about physiological loss of control. But it was easier and more attention-getting for readers and the popular press to quote the passage in which Jellinek speaks of loss of control quite flatly as "that stage . . . when the ingestion of one alcoholic drink sets up a chain reaction so that [alcoholics] are unable to adhere to their intention 'to have one or two drinks only' but continue to ingest more and more . . . contrary to their volition."[13] This dramatic statement, however, happens to be a passage in which Jellinek was not speaking for himself but was reporting to his readers the claims of A.A. Though on occasion Jellinek put the matter in this way, usually he was more cautious and qualified.[14]

Yet out-of-context quotations of statements made by A.A. members took on a new authority because Jellinek had cited them. Despite his own scholarly reservations and nuances, his work had the practical effect of reinforcing the A.A. colloquial axiom, "one drink, one drunk" and of encouraging people to speak of alcoholics as driven to drink by an "overwhelming desire," an "irresistible craving," or a "compulsion." Thus the "folk science" of alcoholism was propagated.[15]

But more important than the unappreciated scholarly nuances or popular exaggerations, it was the inadequacy of Jellinek's data that caused much of his classic work to fail the test of later scientific scrutiny. For all of Jellinek's findings and hypotheses, all his charts, diagrams, and statistics were based on data obtained from A.A. members. Jellinek worked from questionnaires that A.A. had designed and distributed through its membership newsletter, *The Grapevine*. Jellinek's own caution about the limitations of his data is reflected in his noting that the questions were not adequate and that "essential categories" were lacking. We must add that at that time A.A. was still a relatively small, self-selected group.

In sum, Jellinek's highly influential articles were based on questionnaires completed by 98 male members of A.A. Of the 158 questionnaires returned, Jellinek had eliminated 60, excluding the data from some A.A. members who had pooled and averaged their answers on a single questionnaire because they shared their newsletter. Jellinek also excluded all questionnaires filled out by women because their answers differed greatly from the men's. No wonder Jellinek spoke of the limitations of the data. And no wonder his data conformed so closely to the A.A. model. Even in 1960, Jellinek acknowledged the lack of any demonstrated scientific foundation for his proposals. Of the lack of evidence he remarked, "For the time being this may suffice, but not indefinitely." [16]

In the late 1960s national surveys of heavy drinking began to appear that contradicted the sequence of phases described by Jellinek.[17] Many people had problems with drinking, yet they reported no loss of control. Others claimed they experienced loss of control but reported that they had no problems with police, family, finances, employment, auto accidents, or social life. Such alcohol-related problems are now known to come and go in a wide variety of patterns: they do not cluster in any regular way, do not emerge in any uniform sequence, and do not show up at all in the lives of many heavy drinkers. Important, too, is the fact that many drinkers with numerous and severe problems "mature out" of trouble. The descent to the "bottom" is not inevitable, and a return from heavy drinking to moderation is common.[18]

In the scientific community, then, Jellinek's hypothesis of

alcoholism as a disease with a unique sequence of stages and a regular pattern of symptoms has failed to receive general assent: "[Jellinek's] concept of a natural progression of the symptoms underlying the 'disease' of gamma alcoholism endured for many years. In the past decade, however, there has appeared a compelling and coherent body of empirical work that contradicts belief in the orderly evolution of alcoholism."[19]

Although no scientists in the field accept the classic disease concept, proper scientific differences of opinion do remain about the relevance of the term *disease* to some forms of chronic heavy drinking. We will examine these controversies in detail in Chapters 2 and 3. For now, it is sufficient to note that much of the debate concerns a semantic argument about competing definitions of the word *disease* as applied to behaviors that have some biological determinants. No one in the debate is seeking to resurrect the classic disease concept.

## The Politics of Alcoholism

Unfortunately, the wealth of new and better studies that have soundly refuted the classic disease concept have so far had little influence on the general public. Almost everyone outside the scientific community still takes it for gospel that there is a scientifically proven, uniquely patterned drinking history peculiar to a disease called alcoholism. And despite the scientific evidence, the classic disease concept has been assiduously promoted by a variety of interest groups in the public and private sectors.

I do not mean to imply that there has been a malign conspiracy to suppress evidence. But political and economic pressures as well as various constituencies within the health-services field have played a powerful role in actively promoting the scientifically discredited classic disease concept.

In the past ten years the treatment of alcoholism has be-

come a very big business. Each year over $1 billion in tax reve-
nues and health-insurance coverage is spent on inpatient and
outpatient alcoholism treatment programs run by public and
private hospitals and health-services centers. To ensure continued public support and funding, the alcoholism treatment
programs have formed national, state, and local umbrella organizations that publicize their efforts and lobby elected offi-
cials and influential citizens. From the National Council on
Alcoholism on down, these politically oriented organizations
form a truly powerful and ubiquitous pressure group. And
because the majority of the treatment programs are based on
the disease concept of alcoholism, their lobbying, public relations, and advertising efforts inevitably propagate the disease
theme.[20]

How can it be that the very treatment programs themselves
are working from the scientifically untenable disease concept? One key factor is the widespread presence in the treatment and lobbying communities of paraprofessional staff
members who define themselves as "recovering alcoholics."
Indeed, the largest single category of direct service staff in
programs specifically concerned with alcohol consists of counselors without professional degrees,[21] many of whom were
once heavy drinkers and now claim special qualification to
help others by reason of their own experience. Since their
own treatment was effected at a time when the classic disease
concept of alcoholism was dominant, they tend to have faith
in the old dogma and tend to perceive any challenge to the
disease concept as a challenge to the validity of their own
emotional ordeal and conversion to sobriety.

Furthermore, because this group of service staff has not
had the benefit of scientific or professional training, they tend
to be—like most people who are not scientists—relatively un-
concerned about the issue of scientific validity. In all sincerity
they believe that the experiences and anecdotal information
they offer as evidence for their beliefs constitute proof posi-

tive of their claims. Even as they reject genuinely scientific analysis as quibbling, they also insist that their doctrine is medically correct and scientific. In effect, within the treatment programs there is an ongoing internecine battle between experiential and scientific approaches to alcohol abuse:

> The field of alcoholism has long been manned by paraprofessionals. They look on the influx of scientific professionals with some concern. If the paraprofessionals were to desert the field, most programs would grind to a halt; however, the lack of professionals would have only a modest impact. Thus the field of treatment is dominated by paraprofessional values, attitudes, and concepts. This is leading to an ideological conflict between the established paraprofessional approach to treatment and new scientific approaches to treatment. . . .
>
> Paraprofessionals often see empirical scientific data as obscure, irrelevant, or contradictory to their personal experiential knowledge of alcoholism.[22]

Why haven't we heard more from the scientists and researchers about this strife? Intimidation should not be discounted. The classic disease concept remains the cornerstone of traditional treatment and public opinion, the central premise of media coverage and social debate, such that anyone who publicly doubts or challenges the disease concept is likely to be ignored, dismissed, or ostracized. In this version of the emperor's new clothes, truthfulness can threaten, block, or ruin the truthteller's career.

A second factor is that all program staff, paraprofessionals and professionals, have a stake in their organizations' financial survival. So in turn they have a stake in persuading government, private funders, and potential clients and families of the truth of the organizational doctrine. With the dramatic increase in competition among public and privately operated programs (which are expected to generate revenues to cover deficits in other departments of the sponsoring hospitals and health organizations), the courting of potential clients has become particularly intense. Major advertising campaigns on

TV and in the newspapers only reinforce the disease concept in the public's mind.

The economic factor is also powerful for researchers, who need major funding for complex long-term clinical studies. The royal road to public support and funding for research in contemporary American political life is the claim that the work bears on public health and the conquest of disease. Researchers whose work falls under a medical category are most likely to receive sustained major support.

Thus the public relations and advertising undertaken by the treatment lobby serves the research community's ends by authenticating, at least in the public's mind, the claim that alcoholism research is medical research and therefore entitled to its share of government and foundation funds.

## Misleading the Public for Its Own Good

Another important influence on the public conduct of scientists is the concern that revealing the bankruptcy of the classic disease concept might discourage heavy drinkers from seeking help. The essence of this rationale is that if chronic drinkers are told that there is no disease of alcoholism, they will see their drinking as a personal failing; out of guilt and shame, they will tend to hide or deny their problems. But however well-intentioned, this line of thinking can confuse the issue for the public. When scientists use the word *disease* in regard to alcoholism, the public naturally assumes that decisive scientific evidence justifies the usage.

In technical publications unread by the general public, at least several scientists have discussed the social utility of classifying alcohol abuse as a disease:

> In specific circumstances it may be desirable for sociocultural, legal, political, and therapeutic goals to label alcohol dependence

as a "disease," perhaps especially at the time of acute physical symptomatology. At the same time the alcohol-dependent person may appropriately be labeled as "sick." Such circumstances should be carefully delineated and limited in application to specific situations.

To have persuaded society to shift a particular type of deviancy from the bad role to the sick role could . . . whatever the logic, whatever the science, prove to be an event of importance.

The decision as to when a syndrome is to be designated a disease is in large measure socially determined and must be congruent with wider cultural interests and habits.

Calling alcoholism a disease, rather than a behavior disorder, is a useful device both to persuade the alcoholic to admit his alcoholism and to provide a ticket for admission into the health care system. I willingly concede, however, that alcohol dependence lies on a continuum and that in scientific terms *behavior disorder* will often be a happier semantic choice than *disease*.[23]

Such tactics are proposed with good intentions. But to invoke the mantle of science in this way, no matter how worthy the social goals, ultimately is a disservice, for it prevents the public from engaging in a free and open debate of truly controversial issues that involve millions of persons and billions of dollars.

It is true that some researchers offer bona fide scientific reasons for continuing to characterize some heavy drinking as a specific disease, alcoholism. But, as we will see in subsequent chapters, the concept of alcoholism they have in mind is very different from the classic concept; indeed it is at best a highly attenuated notion of disease.

## Other Motives and Other Players

The liquor industry is another player in this story of how and why the classic disease concept of alcoholism continues to be promoted and endorsed in the public arena. The classic disease concept admirably suits the interests of the liquor industry: By acknowledging that a small minority of the drinking population is susceptible to the disease of alcoholism, the industry can implicitly assure consumers that the vast majority of people who drink are *not* at risk. This compromise is far preferable to both the old temperance commitment to prohibition, which criminalized the entire liquor industry, and to newer approaches that look beyond the small group diagnosable as alcoholics to focus on the much larger group of heavy drinkers who develop serious physical, emotional, and social problems.

The final major player in this charade, though largely passive in its role, is the general public. We are a people who for the most part do not understand but profoundly trust the sophisticated technology and science that produce daily miracles for us. So the prospect of a single medical "breakthrough" that will provide the physical remedy for a specific disease of alcoholism is both plausible and welcome.[24] We resist the idea that there is no single remedy to heavy drinking. We prefer not to hear that *heavy drinking* and *alcoholism* are merely labels that cover a variety of social and personal problems caused by the interplay of many poorly understood physiological, psychological, social, and cultural factors.

Our hunger for technical breakthroughs is readily fed by the hand of those who promote the classic disease concept. For decades newspapers, magazines, and TV shows have been reporting that one or another group of researchers appears to be on the verge of discovering *the* cause or *the* cure for alcoholism. But it is a kind of intellectual pyramid scheme. Before the public has had a chance to realize that the promised breakthrough has not been confirmed, a new breakthrough appears on the horizon.

In 1985, for example, the *New York Times Magazine* featured a lengthy article entitled "A New Attack on Alcoholism."[25]

True to form, the reporter announced that "scientists appear to be on the verge of exciting breakthroughs," acknowledged that the research is "still in the experimental stage," and conveyed the scientists' "hope" that important results will accrue. The columns of impressive technical detail were punctuated by qualifiers that alerted more conscientious readers to the fact that they were being served up the latest in well-educated speculation and optimism, not scientifically confirmed truth. The promise of a "new attack" ever reassures us that progress is being made, and it reinforces our faith that medical technology will save us.

## Conclusions

Such, then, in brief compass, is the story of how we as a society have come to believe in the convenient fiction of the classic disease concept. It is a remarkable story, and a disturbing one. No one has plotted an evil conspiracy to keep vital information secret; no one has censored information—indeed, the scientific literature fills bookshelves. Yet to all intents and purposes, the general public has been poorly informed, misinformed, and misled. Constructs formed on the basis of social and political ideologies have been repeated so many times that we take them as self-evident truths.[26] Data that refute the creed are ignored, condemned, or spurned as nonsense or heresy. More than once when I've lectured about the scientific facts about alcohol abuse, I've been told by listeners, "Though these things may be true, you shouldn't spread the word because it will shake people's faith in a useful lie." But hiding our heads in the sand or repeating folkloric formulas certainly is not the best we can do, as individuals or as a society, to respond to the personal, medical, social, and economic consequences of alcohol abuse.

# Notes

1. Cited in Rorabaugh, *The Alcoholic Republic* (1979), 30. On colonial attitudes, see also Hunt, "Spirits of the Colonial Economy" (1987), and Levine, "The Good Creature of God and the Demon Rum" (1981). On earlier attitudes, see Austin and Prendergast, "Chronology of Alcohol Use and Controls" (1987).

2. See Rorabaugh (1979), 25; Levine (1981).

3. Rorabaugh (1979), 48.

4. Levine (1981), 116.

5. For consumption data, see Rorabaugh (1979), 8–10; Moser, *Prevention of Alcohol-Related Problems* (1980), 53; Room, "Measurement and Distribution of Drinking Patterns and Problems in General Populations" (1977), 80.

6. See Levine (1981); Rorabaugh (1979), 26; Levine, "The Discovery of Addiction" (1978).

7. Levine (1978), 151; Rorabaugh (1979), 39–42.

8. Quoted in Bernard, "From the Fast Day Sermon to the Temperance Address" (1984), 12.

9. For a classic account of the temperance movement, see Gusfield, *Symbolic Crusade* (1963).

10. For a brief history of Alcoholics Anonymous, see Rudy, *Becoming Alcoholic* (1986), 7–12; Robinson, *Talking Out of Alcoholism* (1979), 15–16.

11. Mann, *Primer on Alcoholism* (1950), 15–16. Mann's book is one of the classic texts used by A.A.

12. Jellinek, "Phases in the Drinking History of Alcoholics" (1946) and "The Phases of Alcohol Addiction" (1952).

13. Jellinek, *The Disease Concept of Alcoholism* (1960), 41.

14. See Keller, "On the Loss-of-Control Phenomenon in Alcoholism" (1972), 157.

15. Pattison, "Ten Years of Change in Alcoholism Treatment Findings" (1977), 262. Rodin, "Alcoholism as a Folk Disease" (1981).

16. Jellinek (1960), 159.

17. See especially Cahalan and Room, *Problem Drinking Among American Men* (1974), and also Cahalan, "Subcultural Differences in Drinking Behavior in U.S. National Surveys" (1978).

18. Rohan, "Comments on the NCA Criteria Study" (1978), 215; Clark and Cahalan, "Changes in Problem Drinking over a Four-Year Span" (1976), 258. For a review of the accumulation of evidence disconfirming Jellinek's model, see Rudy (1986).

19. Vaillant, "The Contribution of Prospective Studies in the Understanding of Etiologic Factors in Alcoholism" (1984), 279. See Polich and Kaelber, "Sample Surveys and the Epidemiology of Alcoholism" (1985), 72.

20. For a full-scale study of the treatment lobby, see Wiener, *The Politics of Alcoholism* (1981); see also Olson and Gerstein, *Alcohol in America* (1985), 8–9; Room, "Treatment-Seeking Populations and Larger Realities" (1980), 216–17.

21. Saxe et al., "The Effectiveness and Costs of Alcoholism Treatment" (1983), 31.

22. Pattison, Sobell, and Sobell, *Emerging Concepts of Alcohol Dependence* (1977), 262.

23. The four sources quoted are Pattison, "The Selection of Treatment Modalities for the Alcoholic Patient" (1985), 192; Edwards, "The Status of Alcoholism as a Disease" (1970), 161; Edwards et al., *Alcohol-Related Disabilities* (1977), 9; and Vaillant, *The Natural History of Alcoholism* (1983), 20.

24. On the theme of the "medicalization" of alcohol problems and its role in imposing social control over "sick" individuals, see Room, "Sociological Aspects of the Disease Concept of Alcoholism" (1983), 76–80; Mäkela, "What Can Medicine Properly Take On?" (1980); and Levine (1978).

25. Franks, "A New Attack on Alcoholism" (1985), 47.

26. On the transformation of social symbols into apparent objective realities, see Gusfield, *The Culture of Public Problems* (1981); Wiener (1981); Levine (1978); Room, *Governing Images of Alcohol and Drug Problems* (1978).

CHAPTER 2

# Can Alcoholics Control
# Their Drinking?

In this chapter I want to focus on the central premise of the classic disease concept of alcoholism, loss of control. The classic disease concept proposes a simple hypothesis: Chronic heavy drinkers do not stop or limit their drinking—despite the medical, emotional, social, and financial problems they may encounter—because they *cannot* control their drinking, even when they realize that it would be prudent or preferable for them to do so.

According to the classic doctrine, the breakdown of a drinker's self-control mechanism is the key symptom of the disease of alcoholism. Or, as one of the A.A. primers puts it: "Alcoholism is a disease which manifests itself chiefly by the uncontrollable drinking of the victim, who is known as an alcoholic."[1] In keeping with this definition of the problem, the first of the twelve steps of A.A. teaching requires drinkers to confess their lack of control: "We admitted that we were powerless over alcohol—that our lives had become unmanageable."

31

As we will see, the consensus among researchers today is to reject the classic idea of an alcohol-induced inability to control drinking. Some researchers reject the entire notion outright. Others use the phrase "loss of control," but they proffer highly attenuated (and dubiously scientific) definitions of the phenomenon. In order to understand the significance of the current debate, we need to review the classic notion of loss of control and explore the sorts of evidence that have scientifically discredited this still-popular cliché.

## What Is Meant by "Loss of Control"?

Anyone who has ever observed the behavior of a chronic heavy drinker cannot help feeling a sense of powerful momentum at work. In some way the inclination to down another drink seems to escape the full reach of rational judgment and of cool and deliberate free choice. While all observers, both professionals and laypersons, have noted this momentum, its particular power—its strength, nature, and origin—remains a subject of debate. Advocates of the classic disease concept, for example, speak of alcohol as a dominating necessity for the alcohol-dependent person. A.A. theory posits that the alcoholic's ability to control his or her conduct in regard to drink is destroyed by a bodily malfunction. Just as someone with a cold cannot stop sneezing, or someone with nerve damage cannot control a paralyzed limb, alcoholics cannot voluntarily control their drinking behavior. In this view, alcoholics are victims of physiological and neurological abnormalities that cause uncontrollable behavior.

As we noted in Chapter 1, Jellinek's earliest papers seemed to confirm this picture. But by 1960 Jellinek had distinguished two distinct forms of loss of control.[2] In what he called delta alcoholism, drinkers have no control over whether or not to drink, and they drink all day, every day, though usually with control enough over the amount to avoid becoming grossly intoxicated. This delta pattern was intended to describe the habits of the traditional French wine-drinker. The gamma pattern, though, was the one that Jellinek saw as characteristic of Americans. The gamma drinker's first drink is voluntary, but once ingested it triggers a loss of control and the drinker is unable to refrain from continuing to drink, so long as liquor is available, until feeling too sick or too drunk to continue. This gamma loss of control is the essence of what Jellinek had originally labeled "alcohol addiction," though in his more cautious moments he explained that loss of control did not mean that uncontrollable drinking was inevitable, only that it was very likely to occur.

In sum, the disease of gamma alcoholism was alleged to cause the drinker to experience a physiologically based loss of control over drinking, an irresistible or overwhelming compulsion to drink once he had opened the gate by having one drink. But almost immediately after Jellinek proposed this theory, he and other responsible researchers began to qualify and revise the formulation. Everyone who worked with alcohol abusers admitted that "One drink away from a drunk" was just a slogan used by A.A., but not a literal truth. Mark Keller, who was an early colleague of Jellinek's at Yale and has himself become an influential figure in alcoholism studies, explained:

> What is fascinating about that slogan is that nearly all the alcoholics I have known, including those who in all sincerity proclaim that slogan, have told me that, even during the course of the severest stage of their active alcoholism, they had a drink or two or three on many occasions and stopped without further drinking, until on some other occasion, days or weeks later, they did not stop. Some could take a drink or two daily for days or weeks without going off on a bout.[3]

Furthermore, Jellinek's gamma alcoholism posed a contradiction for treatment programs. If the loss of control is triggered by the first drink, then the only hope for an alcoholic is to refrain from that first drink, that is, total abstention. But if loss of control is triggered only *after* the first drink, and not before, why should the alcoholic have any special difficulty mustering the self-control to simply avoid that first drink? Why should abstinence pose any special problem? In a lengthy discussion of the matter years after Jellinek enunciated the concept of gamma alcoholism, Keller acknowledged this fundamental inconsistency and insisted that either loss of control had to exist prior to the first drink or else there could be no disease such as gamma alcoholism.[4]

## Do Alcoholics Really Lack Control?

Even while the public and many courts have come to accept the classic idea of loss of control as the central fact that explains chronic heavy drinking, researchers have been publishing decisive evidence disproving the myth.[5]

Beginning in the 1960s various experimental programs were initiated to test the loss-of-control conjecture and to establish more accurately the patterns of drinking and control that chronic drinkers exhibit. One early major series of such studies broke the treatment taboo by allowing alcoholics to drink during their hospital stays; other researchers soon did likewise.[6]

In one classic experiment, the subjects were allowed to perform a trivially simple task (repeatedly pressing a button according to instructions) that would earn them credit toward measured amounts of alcohol. These subjects were accustomed to drinking a quart of whiskey a day, and they suffered withdrawal when they stopped. During the experiment they could earn an ounce of bourbon in anywhere from five to fifteen minutes, depending on their speed in pushing the button. Though the task was monotonous, they could also watch TV, eat, or talk at the same time. The amount of bourbon served and the timing of it were up to the drinker.

The subjects participated for one or two months, and at any time they could have earned enough to drink to become totally intoxicated. But in all the variations of the experiments, according to one cautious summary, "none of the subjects . . . attempted in a situation where they could determine the volume and pattern of their own drinking to drink themselves into a state of unconsciousness or collapse." Moreover, the subjects actually demonstrated control over their drinking, in that:

> (i) they drank to maintain high but roughly constant BAC's [blood alcohol content] during shorter drinking periods; (ii) they did not drink continuously but spontaneously initiated and terminated drinking sessions over a longer experimental period; (iii) they tended to work for and drink moderate amounts of alcohol and did not consume it as soon as it became available; (iv) some subjects chose to taper off their drinking in order to avoid or reduce withdrawal symptoms following termination of the experiment; and (v) subjects chose to work over one- or two-day periods [without drinking] to accumulate alcohol rather than to drink to abolish partial withdrawal symptoms.

From the experiments, the researchers could only conclude that "All these observations are inconsistent with the concept of loss of control in the sense of an inability to stop once drinking has commenced, and with the related concept of craving in the sense of an uncontrollable urge to consume more and more alcohol during a drinking session."[7]

The researchers also found that the amount of alcohol consumed by their subjects was "a function of the cost of alcohol, measured by the degree of effort required to obtain it."[8] In other words, individuals' patterns of drinking were found to depend significantly on the costs and benefits *perceived by the drinker*—an observation that radically contradicts the idea of some overpowering inner drive that completely overwhelms all reason or choice. That drinking patterns are shaped by considerations of cost, convenience, benefits, or deprivations has been demonstrated in a number of other studies as well. One research team was able, by offering small payments, to get alcoholics to voluntarily abstain from drink even though drink was available, or to moderate their drinking voluntarily even after an initial "priming dose" of liquor had been consumed.[9] (The larger the "priming dose," the less moderate the subsequent drinking, until a modest increase in the amount of payment offered prompted a resumption of moderation.)

In another experiment, drinkers were willing to do a limited amount of boring work (pushing a lever) in order to earn a drink, but when the "cost" of a drink rose (that is, more lever pushing was asked of them) they were unwilling to "pay" the higher price. Still another experiment allowed alcoholic patients access to up to a fifth of liquor, but subjects were told that if they drank more than five ounces they would be removed from the pleasant social environment they were in. Result: Most of the time subjects limited themselves to moderate drinking.[10]

During the 1970s the evidence continued to mount. In 1972 an evaluation of a series of seven independent studies concluded that researchers "consistently reported no findings of phenomena such as physiological or psychological craving for further alcohol as a result of initial inebriation." And in 1977 a review of the scientific literature cited nearly sixty pertinent reports of experiments and clinical studies and concluded that "within a hospital or laboratory environment, the drinking of chronic alcoholics is explicitly a function of environmental contingencies."[11] The reviewers noted that the subjects were able to control their consumption on their own and also when they were "rewarded" for doing so by special privileges, opportunities for socialization, or money.

True, these results were all obtained in special environments (hospitals) with alcoholics who were often receiving special support and help. But if these drinkers were able to control their drinking in these special settings, one of two explanations must hold. Either (1) the careful observers in the special settings are noticing behaviors that careful observers would also detect in everyday situations or (2) the change in setting from home to hospital indeed radically affects alcoholics' self-control and drinking patterns.

Either of these explanations undermines the classic loss-of-control conjecture. If the first explanation holds, then loss of control is a stereotype born of faulty observation and a misunderstanding of drinkers' behavior. If the second explanation holds, then it is the social setting, not any chemical effect of alcohol, that influences drinkers' abilities to exert control over their drinking.

More broadly, in all these experiments the subjects' behavior exemplifies the general principles of human motivation that we all recognize. Given what they perceive as substantial reasons to limit their drinking—money, sociability, privileges, or conveniences—these drinkers do limit their drinking. In these special settings, a drinker's self-control may also be reinforced by the *absence* of situations that prompt drinking at home, such as domestic or social frustrations, social enticements, or job anxieties. But clearly it is each drinker's perception of the pattern of positive and negative motivations, and not an uncontrollable abnormal chemical-physiological reaction, that decisively affects the choice to drink, to abstain, or to drink in moderation.

The reason that this element of choice has so often escaped notice is that the chronic drinker's perception of the advantages and disadvantages of drinking on a particular occasion—the weight the drinker assigns to the pros and cons— may often appear irrational to the detached observer. The drinker's fears and anxieties, his sense of the consequences of certain choices, may be quite different or far more emotionally intense than the observer's. But although the drinker's anxieties may appear irrational, the choice to drink may be an intelligible attempt to deflect those anxieties. To the outside observer, however, it is the visible behavior—the drinking—rather than the drinker's anxiety that seems utterly irrational.[12]

If we move from experiments conducted in special settings to real-life observation, we find the same principles at work. The consensus in the research literature is that even in their normal, everyday settings, chronic heavy drinkers often moderate their drinking or abstain voluntarily, the choice depending on their perceptions of the costs and benefits. For example, in one court trial that I studied the defendant was a diagnosed alcoholic who was already on probation for drunk driving. While on probation he had regularly reported to his probation officer, who testified that the defendant always arrived sober, despite the fact that, as ample testimony from others revealed, he had not curtailed his overall drinking during the period in question. At the time he was running a prosperous business and had every motive to stay out of jail. So he simply stopped drinking whenever the time to report approached.[13]

This sensible self-control by a diagnosed alcoholic is not an unusual phenomenon. Many people who fit the alcoholic profile go through periods of extremely moderate use or abstinence: "In any given month, one half of alcoholics will be abstinent, with a mean of four months of being dry in any one-year to two-year period."[14] Convincing anecdotal evidence repeatedly shows that alcoholics choose to moderate or abstain for reasons that are important *to them*.[15]

Several recent general arguments still defend versions of loss of control, contending that the experiments and studies of the sort just discussed may not have used "true" alcoholics. Yet many of the subjects in these experiments were diagnosed alcoholics. In over eighty studies in the past decade that report on alcoholics who return to some moderated form of drinking, at least half the subjects were diagnosed as gamma alcoholics. In the face of this evidence, the question of whether the subjects were "true" alcoholics seems a mere polemical device, not a sustainable objection to the conduct of the experiments.


## What Role Does Alcohol Play in Triggering Sustained Drinking?

Another attack on the classic loss-of-control hypothesis is based on experiments that demonstrate that an alcoholic's drinking behavior is influenced by such factors as the drinker's subjective expectations or the social setting of the drinking.

In one landmark experiment, the alcoholic subjects were divided into four groups. Members of each group were asked to compare and "taste-rate" three different brands of a beverage and were told that they could drink as much as they wanted from each of three large pitchers. One group was led to believe that they were being offered three brands of a vodka-tonic beverage, although in fact all three pitchers had pure tonic water. The second group was led to believe that their beverages were all brands of pure tonic water, although in fact each pitcher contained a mixture of vodka and tonic. The third group was given pure tonic, the fourth group the vodka-tonic mix, but both of these groups were told the truth about their beverages. The subjects were left alone to sample as much or as little as they chose. In this way the experimenters hoped to observe whether the amount that these alcoholic subjects drank was related to how much alcohol they actually drank or to how much alcohol they *thought* they were drinking.[16]

The results form a consistent pattern. The subjects who

were truthfully told that their pitchers contained only tonic water drank the least. They drank only enough to taste-rate, but no more. A significantly greater quantity of the beverages was drunk by those subjects who were truthfully told that their pitchers had vodka and tonic.

The interesting twist is that the behavior of the two groups who were misled about their beverages depended on what they believed they were drinking and not on the drink itself. The subjects who mistakenly thought they were drinking pure tonic drank just about as little as the drinkers who did receive plain tonic. And the subjects who mistakenly thought they were drinking alcohol drank just about as much as the drinkers who did receive alcohol. Thus, for these alcoholics, it was their beliefs about what they were drinking, not the actual alcohol content of the drink, that prompted heavier drinking.

Similar results have been obtained in other experiments, disproving the myth that the ingestion of alcohol biochemically triggers additional alcohol consumption by chronic drinkers. Quite to the contrary, as these experiments show, it is the drinker's mind-set, the drinker's beliefs and attitudes about alcohol, that influence the level of consumption.[17]

It has been argued that such experiments are faulty because the priming dose (the initial drink alleged to trigger loss of control) is often only the equivalent of a drink or two, a small amount for a heavy drinker. But since the classic disease concept hinges on the premise that it takes only one drink to trigger loss of control, that after one drink the alcoholic *can't* stop himself, these experiments with a priming dose equal to a drink or two are exactly pertinent.

Similarly, it has been argued that these experiments are not realistic because the eventual total amount drunk by many of the subjects was relatively moderate for an alcoholic. But since all the subjects had free access to additional liquor, the moderation was due to self-control, to the subjects' choice not to drink more. Whether because of specific incentives to limit their drinking, the absence of factors that usually triggered their drinking at home, or their mistaken belief about what they were drinking—these diagnosed alcoholics showed no signs of uncontrollable drinking.

## "Craving"

At various points, versions of the disease concept have suggested "craving" as the biochemical or psychological mechanism that prompts heavy sustained drinking. It has been proposed that alcoholics at times experience an irresistible physical desire for alcohol, a desire so intense and powerful that no amount of reasoning or willpower can defeat their thirst for alcohol. This definition of *craving* has been criticized by various writers as an empty notion, a semantic trick or a pseudo-explanation.[18] For this definition only leads us in circles. Whenever an alcoholic drinks in a grossly excessive manner, one can say it is an instance of loss of control caused by craving. But whenever an alcoholic doesn't drink or drinks moderately, one can only say there was on that occasion no craving. Since there is no independent way of deciding whether craving is or isn't present, the word becomes a synonym for—not an explanation of—excessive drinking.

Some recent experiments have reported bona fide independent evidence that alcohol consumption does generate a heavy drinker's craving for more alcohol.[19] But in these studies *craving* does not mean "an irresistible desire." In one study, for example, alcoholics were asked whether they experienced a strong or a mild craving for alcohol. Here, however, the modifier "mild" defeats the idea of urgency in the concept of craving, suggesting a desire hardly so irresistible as to overwhelm all other considerations. Furthermore, asking such a question of an alcoholic who has been taught that "addicts" have a "craving" for the substance they are "addicted to" seems to prejudice the results, especially since *craving* was not carefully defined for the interviewees in these studies. Not much, in sum, can be learned by asking chronic heavy drinkers if they ever have urges, strong or weak, to have a drink. Once *craving* is redefined to exclude the notion of an irresistible desire, it cannot serve as the key to the classic concept of loss of control.

Other studies have retained the meaning of *craving* as an intense desire and report a correlation between craving and drinking and a correlation between craving and physical withdrawal symptoms.[20] The first correlation, that drinkers express a strong desire to drink prior to or during the act of drinking, is hardly surprising and even tautological, telling us that people who frequently drink heavily often have a strong desire to drink. As to the second correlation, we have already reviewed experimental evidence that shows that alcoholics often enough do not drink even when experiencing withdrawal distress. Thus even if some drinkers report having felt a craving for alcohol during withdrawal, the clinical observations show that chronic drinkers often resist this craving and abstain or drink in moderation even as they are feeling withdrawal distress. That is, whatever feelings of craving were reported by one group, the behavior of the other group shows that the craving was far from irresistible.

Several other advocates of the craving hypothesis present data that actually undermine their point. For example, one researcher approvingly quotes a study reporting that alcoholics given initial priming drinks exhibit a very much higher correlation of craving and drinking when they are in a conducive setting (bar-type atmosphere, peanuts, liquor bottles, etc.) than when they are in a nonconducive one (antiseptic-smelling lab).[21] These craving effects were achieved even when subjects were given a placebo primer, that is, a beverage that had only a tiny bit of liquor floated on the surface to provide the liquor taste. In the conducive setting, the faked drink was followed by a high degree of craving. Whatever *craving* may mean in this context, the lesson to be learned here is that the desire reflects crucially the social and psychological setting, and need not be a direct chemical result of consuming alcohol.

Still other attempts to measure craving have relied on more objective signs such as hand tremors and increased rate of drinking, rather than on self-report. Although measuring these behaviors lends a new air of objectivity to the search, hand tremors and rate of drinking are not equivalent to the classical notion of craving. No one denies the existence of withdrawal symptoms such as hand tremors, but it is a long leap from observing hand tremors to deducing an irresistible desire. And certainly hand tremors do not cause chronic drinking, nor are they even inevitably a side-effect of it.

Craving, then, is another myth.

## Revisions of the Disease Concept

One extremely influential voice in the field of alcoholism studies is that of George Vaillant, a scientist of long experience, now working at Harvard University. Vaillant still advocates characterizing alcoholism as a disease but, like many other contemporary researchers, his view differs markedly from the classic disease concept. Vaillant has been persuaded by the experimental and clinical studies that "in a laboratory setting, confirmed alcoholics can drink with moderation" and that "the concept of loss of the capacity for controlled drinking is, at best, a relative concept."[22] Vaillant also acknowledges that an alcoholic's control over drinking is influenced by psychological factors and social setting, and that experiments confirm that "alcoholics can be successfully taught to return to social drinking in the community."

Another influential group of research and clinical authorities who also support a highly modified disease concept of alcoholism reject the classic stereotype in these words: "the person suffering from [the alcohol-dependence syndrome] is not an automaton in the grip of an all-controlling and pathological process which totally denies his self-responsibility."[23]

A series of attempts have been made to salvage something from the classic loss-of-control hypothesis. Since drinking is not automatically triggered when alcohol enters the system of diagnosed alcoholics, it has been suggested that what is at issue is "inconsistency of control of drinking," or that loss of control is "relative and variable" as well as "multifactorial" (that is, it depends on social and psychological as well as biological factors).[24]

In Mark Keller's widely cited revision of the loss-of-control concept, he affirms that loss of control is not inevitable, but "if an alcoholic takes a drink, he can never be sure he will be able to stop."[25] Keller also posits that the disease, and therefore the loss of control, can go into temporary remission for periods of varying length or even indefinitely.

This new approach to loss of control so emasculates the concept that it becomes useless in explaining or predicting drinking behavior. There is indeed a phenomenon involving the strong inclination to drink to excess, and it does need to be made intelligible if possible. But the attempt to account for this by reference to an on-again, off-again loss of control that follows no discernible pattern will not help anyone understand why heavy drinkers sometimes drink moderately and sometimes go on binges.

## Conclusions

The public has been so indoctrinated by the idea of loss of control that few dare to seem naive by carefully observing alcoholic conduct and acknowledging that heavy drinkers often do moderate and limit their drinking. We may be close to people who have been labeled alcoholics, but we discount our observations of the times they show self-control because we have been told that alcoholics have no control. Or if we do recognize evidence of control, we decide the drinker in question cannot really be a "true" alcoholic. We then minimize or discount that person's drinking problems because the labels "alcoholic" and "disease" don't seem to apply. Both reactions are wrong and unproductive, both in the personal sphere and in the sphere of public health and welfare policy.

Where does this leave us, then, in regard to the idea that heavy drinkers—especially those who have been long-term heavy drinkers—have a hard time controlling their drinking? Let's recapitulate the basic facts that pose the puzzle of the heavy drinker's self-control. On any particular occasion the heavy drinker may drink heavily, or moderately, or may not drink at all, or may start drinking and then voluntarily stop. The choice depends on situational factors (such as the drinker's mood and feelings of frustration, satisfaction, threat) and the social setting. The choice also depends on the rewards or deprivations the drinker believes will ensue, on his or her beliefs about the effects the alcohol will produce, on the cost or inconvenience of obtaining a drink, and so on—all the reasons and motives that affect anyone's decisions about personal conduct. In addition, as we will see in subsequent chapters, the choice depends on cultural, ethnic, religious, regional, and occupational factors, on social class and dynamics, age, and marital status. Thus, on any particular occasion, the drinker's choice will be influenced by the sorts of things that generally influence us all. And yet . . .

And yet when we look beyond any one particular occasion and contemplate the heavy drinker's long-term pattern of conduct, we see that he or she chooses to engage, again and again, in drinking conduct that to most of us seems irrational, imprudent, harmful, and disruptive. We also see that some of these drinkers acknowledge the harm and are plainly in inner conflict; yet they repeatedly choose to drink.

How can we make this combination of facts intelligible and

meaningful, rather than puzzling and paradoxical? We will take up this question in Chapter 5, but first we need to complete the critique of the classic disease concept. The evidence presented in that critique will point us toward the new perspectives we need in order to understand heavy drinking.

## Notes

1. Mann, *Primer on Alcoholism* (1950), 3. On the notion of loss of control, see Armor, "The RAND Reports and the Analysis of Relapse" (1980), 82; Keller, "On the Loss-of-Control Phenomenon in Alcoholism" (1972); Jellinek, "Phases in the Drinking History of Alcoholics" (1946), 28.
2. Jellinek, *The Disease Concept of Alcoholism* (1960), 36–38, 42–44, 145–47.
3. Keller (1972), 156.
4. Keller (1972), 160.
5. An early influential report was Merry, "The 'Loss of Control' Myth" (1966); see also Heather and Robertson, *Controlled Drinking* (1981); Donovan and Marlatt, "Assessment of Expectancies and Behavior Associated with Alcohol Consumption" (1980).
6. The groundbreaking studies are: Mello and Mendelson, "Drinking Patterns During Work-contingent and Non-contingent Alcohol Acquisition" (1972); Mendelson, "Experimentally Induced Chronic Intoxication and Withdrawal in Alcoholics" (1964). See also Gottheil et al., "Fixed-Interval Drinking Decisions" (1972); Cohen et al., "Alcoholism: Controlled Drinking and Incentives for Abstinence" (1971a) and "Moderate Drinking by Chronic Alcoholics" (1971b).
7. The description of this experiment is based on Mello and Mendelson (1972); the summary statements quoted are from Heather and Robertson (1981), 84–85.
8. Heather and Robertson (1981), 85.
9. Cohen et al., 1971(a).
10. The two experiments mentioned in this paragraph are from Bigelow and Liebson, "Cost Factors Controlling Alcoholic Drinking" (1972), and Cohen et al., 1971(b).

11. The two reviews quoted in this paragraph are M. Sobell and L. Sobell, *Individualized Behavior Therapy for Alcoholics* (1972), 1; and Pattison, Sobell, and Sobell, *Emerging Concepts of Alcohol Dependence* (1977), 100.

12. Heather and Robertson (1981), 88–89.

13. Fingarette, "How an Alcoholism Defense Works under the ALI Insanity Test" (1979).

14. Schuckit, *Drug and Alcohol Abuse* (1984), 59.

15. See, for example, Fingarette (1979) and Keller (1972), 156.

16. Marlatt, Deming, and Reid, "Loss of Control Drinking in Alcoholics" (1973).

17. For a recent review of these experiments, see Adesso, "Cognitive Factors in Alcohol and Drug Use" (1985). See also Heather and Robertson (1981), chap. 3; Pattison, Sobell, and Sobell (1977); Maisto, Galizio, and Carey, "Individual Differences in Substance Abuse" (1985); Engle and Williams, "Effect of an Ounce of Vodka on Alcoholics' Desire for Alcohol" (1972).

18. Marlatt, "Craving for Alcohol, Loss of Control, and Relapse" (1978); Mello, "A Semantic Aspect of Alcoholism" (1975).

19. Hodgson, Rankin, and Stockwell, "Craving and Loss of Control" (1978); Ludwig, Wikler, and Stark, "The First Drink" (1974).

20. Hore, *Alcohol Dependence* (1976), 12.

21. Kissin, "The Disease Concept of Alcoholism" (1983), 114, citing Ludwig, Wikler, and Stark (1974).

22. Vaillant, *The Natural History of Alcoholism* (1983), 217–18. Supporting studies cited by Vaillant in this passage are: Paredes et al., "Loss of Control in Alcoholism" (1973); Gottheil et al., "Alcoholics' Patterns of Controlled Drinking" (1973); Mello and Mendelson, "Experimentally Induced Intoxication in Alcoholics" (1970); Merry (1966); Marlatt and Rohsenow, "Cognitive Processes in Alcohol Use" (1980); Hodgson, Rankin, and Stockwell, "Alcohol Dependence and the Priming Effect" (1979).

23. Edwards et al., *Alcohol and Alcoholism* (1979), 55.

24. Hore (1976), 4; Glatt, "The 'Lack of Control' over Alcoholism and Its Implications" (1982), 138–40.

25. Keller (1972), 160.

# CHAPTER 3

# What Causes Alcoholism?

Before the classic disease concept of alcoholism was largely abandoned by scientists, a key question among its proponents was, What is the cause of the disease? This question may now seem pointless inasmuch as we have seen that the heart of the classic disease concept, loss of control, is a confused notion that is contradicted by a bookshelf of experimental evidence. But there is so much misinformation abroad—news of breakthroughs in the discovery of the cause or cure of the disease of alcoholism—that one cannot help wondering if there is some fire where there is so much smoke. If we want to sort out the true from the false, we need to examine the theories about the causes of the so-called disease and also (in the next chapter) the treatments for it.

Despite decades of imminent breakthroughs, the current dominant consensus among researchers is that no single explanation, however complex, has ever been scientifically established as the cause of alcoholism. As one leading research group summarizes the issue: "[the] causes of excessive drinking are always multiple and interactive, and . . . any single-factor model of causation is not only wrong in theory, but in practice will lead to inappropriate responses to the individual, and to imperfect social policies."[1] Nor, as we will soon see, has anyone proposed a scientifically accepted multiple-factor explanation.

## Alcoholism and Alcoholisms

As one begins to read the literature on the causes of alcoholism, one notices that the words *alcoholism* and *alcoholic* have been, and still are, used to mean many different things. Regarding the twin problems of defining alcoholism and determining its cause, a commentator on the diagnostic criteria promulgated by the National Council on Alcoholism (NCA) puts these issues on the table:

> All attempts to identify and define "alcoholism" have failed because the concept itself is fundamentally flawed. "Alcoholism" exists in our language and in our minds, but not in the objective world around us. . . . Like many other attempts to define "alcoholism," the [evaluation of the NCA] criteria and related studies fail because they are based on the erroneous supposition that a unique causal entity exists, which resides within certain alcohol users and somehow motorizes their ingestion behavior. An invisible, underlying factor has been invented and invoked to account for unacceptable drinking. Although this entity remains undiscovered, the observable behavior of drinking and its consequences are interpreted as signs of its existence. This reduces a complex variety of drinking sequences and associated effects to an oversimplified formula which is so widely accepted its denial may seem irresponsible or even absurd. So many words have been written and spoken about "alcoholism" that language alone "confirms" it as a reality.[2]

Much the same vagueness obtains in regard to the word *disease.* In medical texts the word has only a loose, ill-defined allusive sense and is not used as a basis for rigorous scientific discussion. Or in Jellinek's words: "It comes to this, that *a disease is what the medical profession recognizes as such.*"[3]

One reviewer summarizes the broad diversity of theories by noting that "the determination of the underlying causes of alcoholism has been even more intensely debated than its definition" and that "at least three major views of the etiology of alcoholism can be identified: (1) medical, (2) psychological, and (3) sociocultural."[4] Which is a scholar's way of saying that every conceivable perspective has been adopted in trying to explain the causes of alcoholism and none of them has achieved general scientific acceptance. The reviewer then proposes that perhaps a little of each brand of hypothesis is true. So we are left with alcoholism as a disease that is "multiple in origin and complex in development." Instead of a single disease and syndrome (cluster of symptoms), we have a continuum of behaviors ranging from teetotaling to chronic heavy abuse.

The Department of Health, Education and Welfare's publication *Alcohol and Health* epitomizes the consequences of the official inclination to use the term *alcoholism* as though it referred to one definable condition: "The causes of alcoholism are so many and appear in such differing constellations from person to person that one cannot consider treating alcoholism as if it were a single illness with an identifiable and specific etiology, a known course, and a proven response to a particular chemical agent or medical treatment."[5]

Despite the fact that there is no general agreement about the definition of alcoholism, hundreds of hypotheses have been proposed about what causes it. In 1980 a monograph published by the National Institute on Drug Abuse discussed a selection of specially interesting theories—forty-three of them.[6] The temptation to doubt that the theories could all be wrong must be balanced by the thought that, however plausible they may seem, at least most of them must be wrong. After all, how many true explanations can there be?

Thus the best answer we have to the question, What causes the disease of alcoholism? is: There is no such single disease and therefore there is no cause. The very proliferation of widely diverging unsupported hypotheses is not characteristic of solid scientific research. It is characteristic of pseudoscience and faddism.

Obviously, we can consider here only a few of the theories that have been proposed, those that contain the most plausible elements of truth, or are the most widely believed, or the most truly informative from a scientific standpoint. At best any of these theories is only a partial explanation of some aspects of heavy drinking.

## Genetic Hypotheses

Genetic hypotheses have been widely discussed. On crucial points, however, most of the animal and human studies of genetic influences on alcohol abuse are acknowledgedly indecisive.[7] For example, studies of the children of alcoholic parents have shown that these children are statistically at significantly higher than average risk of becoming alcoholics. But this method of study cannot prove that heredity, rather than family environment, is responsible for the increased risk.

Studies of alcoholism in twins have been far more strongly suggestive of a genetic factor.[8] And several skillfully designed studies of adopted children have provided some insights into the nature versus nurture question. Representative of these studies is the pivotal work of Donald W. Goodwin and his associates.[9]

Goodwin's study is based on a simple idea, though one arduous and complex to implement: Find children who were born to an alcoholic mother or father but who were put up for adoption very shortly after birth and thus were not raised by their biological parents; then see whether these children in later life show a higher rate of alcoholism than a comparable group of adopted infants whose biological parents were not alcoholics. Any difference in the rates of alcoholism between the two groups could be attributed to heredity rather than rearing. And since both groups of children were adoptees, any relationship between alcoholism and being an adoptee should be the same for both groups and will, in effect, cancel itself out in comparisons between the two groups.

Goodwin chose to study only male children, and in 85 percent of the cases the biological alcoholic parent was the father. This experimental design followed the lead of earlier studies, which suggested that father-son relationships were likely to show the strongest genetic influence.

The difference in the incidence of alcoholism for Goodwin's two groups was statistically significant. The rate of alcoholism among the adoptees who had an alcoholic biological parent was 3.6 times greater than that among the adoptees whose biological parents were not alcoholics. What added extra persuasiveness to Goodwin's results was that for the subset of sons whose adopting parents happened to be alcoholics, no statistically significant difference was apparent. It was consistently the case that only alcoholism in the biological parents was a statistically significant factor.

Somewhat similar results have been obtained in several other studies.[10] But taken together, these findings do not come anywhere near warranting the conclusion that there is a unique disease of alcoholism which is genetically determined. Besides the question of the differing definitions of *alcoholism* used by the various research teams, at best the studies suggest that heredity is one factor, among many, that pertains in a minority of cases. A second look at the data shows why these qualifications are necessary.

In Goodwin's study, about 18 percent of the sons who had an alcoholic parent became alcoholics, compared to 5 percent of the sons of nonalcoholic parents. The hypothesis is that the difference between these groups is attributable to heredity. But to see the full picture, let's turn the numbers around: 82 percent of the sons who had an alcoholic parent—more than four out of five—did not become alcoholics. So if we generalize from Goodwin's results, we must say that about 80 percent of persons with an alcoholic parent will not become alcoholics. Either the relevant genes are usually not transmitted or the genes are transmitted but are usually outweighed by other factors.

A second implication of Goodwin's study is easier to grasp if we construe a hypothetical example based on a ballpark guess about the percentage of alcoholics in the child-bearing adult population. We have no statistics on this issue, but everyone agrees that many more parents are nonalcoholics than are alcoholics. Let us make a very generous round guess that 10 of 100 child-bearing couples have one alcoholic member and that all 100 couples have two sons each. If 18 percent of the 20 sons born to the couples that have an alcoholic partner go on to become alcoholics, we will have about 4 alcoholic sons in this subset. If 5 percent of the 180 sons born to nonalcoholic parents go on to become alcoholics, we will have 9 alcoholic sons in that subset. That is, only one third of the alcoholic sons will have been born of an alcoholic parent.

Granted these are hypothetical numbers, and the proportions will vary depending on the numbers one picks. But this simple example illustrates how from Goodwin's data we can extrapolate the finding that by far most alcoholics have biological parents who are not themselves alcoholics. When we put this together with our earlier observation that by far most children born of an alcoholic parent will not themselves become alcoholics, we see that any genetic factor must be but one possible factor among others and that this genetic factor makes a difference in only a minority of cases.

I do not want to obscure the practical and scientific importance of the data from genetic studies. People whose parents or siblings are long-term heavy drinkers are "at risk" to some unspecifiable degree. And data on heredity are part of the complex total picture for research scientists. But no one should be misled into thinking that alcoholism is genetic. Not only is such a belief incorrect but also it often leads people to become apathetic or defeatist. It is of the highest practical importance for heavy drinkers and their families and friends to understand that whether a given person becomes a heavy drinker or not is not an issue settled by his or her genes. Even when parents or siblings are heavy drinkers, the fate of a particular person is crucially influenced by conduct, character, beliefs, and environment.

Unfortunately, the significance of genetic factors is in general widely misunderstood. When we see very young children who have an exceptional talent for music or art or foreign languages, we rightly suspect that genes play some significant role. But we don't conclude that each person's social destiny and occupation are rigorously and unalterably determined by his or her genes. Many other circumstances of life and personality combine in infinitely many combinations to shape an individual.

By the same token, as one authority explains, "It is common to find that some genetic contribution can be established for many aspects of human attributes or disorders (ranging from musical ability to duodenal ulcers), and drinking is unlikely to be the exception."[11]

A final important point is that even if genetic factors play a role in some drinking behavior, it does not necessarily follow that they play a role in generating the problem behaviors often associated with heavy drinking. How, for example, could genetic factors explain why almost half of adult males in our country who are heavy drinkers have no drink-related personal or social problems while almost half the adult males in our country who have serious personal and social problems associated with their drinking are not heavy drinkers?[12]

The link between heavy drinking and serious personal and social problems is much looser by far than is generally supposed.[13] And so, even if heavy drinking is in a minority of cases partly ascribable to genetic factors, such factors would not account for differences between problem and nonproblem drinkers.

## Metabolic Hypotheses

We turn now to a group of theories that seek to explain the causes of the supposed disease of alcoholism by looking at human physiology, specifically at the way that our body chemistry reacts to alcohol. The premise is that because of genetic factors or acquired physiological differences, some people's bodies respond to alcohol in an abnormal way that "causes" them to become alcoholics.

One of the physiological hypotheses that made something of a sensation in the 1970s was the proposition that persons who are alcoholics and those identified as at higher than average risk of becoming alcoholics tend to metabolize alcohol in distinctive ways.[14] Some studies measured blood levels of acetaldehyde (an intermediate product in the complex metabolism of alcohol) and reported generally higher levels in alcoholics and alcoholism-prone subjects. But the conjecture that higher acetaldehyde levels somehow produce a physical dependence on alcohol has not been borne out. A review of the literature concludes that "the popular theory that the development of physical dependence upon ethanol [alcohol] is mediated by acetaldehyde is not favored by much experimental evidence."[15]

Other studies have suggested that certain morphinelike substances may be secreted during alcohol metabolism and that these substances significantly affect the way one experiences alcohol intoxication. The facts are so far incomplete; no one has proved that there is a significant difference in the levels of these substances in alcoholics and nonalcoholics: "At present, these findings are only of theoretical interest and will require much more work before their validity can be established."[16] But we can already see that even if a difference were found, it could not account for the drinking patterns of heavy drinkers but only for some aspects of how they experience intoxication. Increased levels of morphinelike substances during the few hours that the body is metabolizing alcohol cannot explain why after a period of sobriety, when the body has been free of alcohol and its metabolic products, an alcoholic will resume heavy drinking.

## Tolerance and Withdrawal

We turn next to what may be the most appealing type of explanation of how people become alcoholics. The various versions of this theory all derive from the fact that long-term heavy drinkers often develop a physical tolerance for alcohol and experience physical withdrawal symptoms when they cease drinking. These physical effects are presumed to produce psychological effects that cause an irresistible craving for alcohol.

A characteristic and widely known version of the theory goes like this: At some point the heavy drinker experiences physical withdrawal symptoms (nervous tension, jitteriness, sweating, and a general feeling of discomfort) when he stops drinking. He discovers that alcohol promptly alleviates these symptoms ("a bit of the hair of the dog"). So he takes a drink and the cycle begins again. Of course, this theory cannot explain why, despite the danger signs, a person continued to drink heavily for a long enough time—it can take years—to develop physical withdrawal symptoms. Nor does it explain why after the drinker has had one or two drinks to alleviate the withdrawal discomfort, he doesn't stop or at least moderate his drinking.

To address these questions, a variation of the theory incorporates an element of operant conditioning, the principle that if a behavior or a response is followed by a reward or benefit (positive reinforcement), a person will be more likely to repeat that behavior or response. Since drinking liquor is followed by a positive feeling—relief of distress—drinking reinforces the tendency to drink. As this conditioning repeats itself, the drinking becomes a stronger and stronger habit. But the drinker's ever more frequent intake of alcohol leads to an increasing physical tolerance for alcohol. That is, it takes more alcohol to achieve the same effect as previously. So, over time, the heavy drinker needs more and more alcohol to obtain relief from withdrawal distress. But drinking greater quantities in turn intensifies the withdrawal symptoms when drinking stops.

The upshot is a vicious cycle: Each successive cessation of drinking induces ever greater withdrawal distress; the drinker must drink ever more alcohol to get relief; the relief, in turn, acts as further reinforcement of the conditioned response of drinking, as well as further increasing tolerance, and further intensifying subsequent withdrawal distress.[17] Ultimately, according to this theory, withdrawal distress becomes so severe that it not only activates the automatic conditioned response of drinking but also induces a fully conscious and desperate craving for alcohol in order to dispel the torture of the withdrawal reaction.

This blend of biochemistry and psychology may be appealing, but several kinds of evidence undermine such explanations of alcoholism by reference to tolerance and withdrawal symptoms.

First, a significant proportion of those drinkers classified as alcoholics do not develop tolerance and withdrawal symptoms. One large-scale study found that 36 percent of diagnosed alcoholics did not have these symptoms, even when they were still drinking regularly.[18] Second, as we saw in Chapter 2, many experiments have shown that alcoholics do not drink while suffering withdrawal distress. The actual behavior of alcoholics simply does not follow the rigid habitual pattern that conditioning theory would lead us to expect.[19] Third, we cannot go along with the assumption that drinking is a positive reinforcement for the alcoholic because it always relieves tension. Clinical observation has revealed that for alcoholics drinking is often not followed by relaxation or euphoria, but frequently by depression or anxiety. As one specialist in the biopsychology of alcoholism says: "We have developed convincing evidence regarding the complexity of alcohol's effect on the emotions, showing that a simplistic reduction of tension does not explain what occurs."[20]

Fourth, laboratory measurements of blood alcohol levels and withdrawal symptoms do not show the relationships that the theories predict. For example, according to the theory, withdrawal symptoms should decrease as blood alcohol levels rise. But this pattern does not regularly occur. Indeed, blood alcohol levels do not uniformly rise relative to the amount of alcohol drunk. Some drinkers can consume as much as a fifth of whiskey a day and still maintain low blood alcohol levels.[21] And the weight of the evidence shows that "alcoholics do not drink consistently to maintain stable blood alcohol levels."[22]

In sum, the phenomena of tolerance and withdrawal symptoms cannot be viewed as *the* cause of alcoholism. The temptation to save the theory by increasingly speculative hypotheses remains strong, however. Some researchers have proposed that subtle residues of physical withdrawal or related bodily conditions may persist as long as six months after severe withdrawal is over, even if abstinence is maintained.[23] But if there were such subtle residues, it is highly implausible to infer that they would produce an irresistible craving that overwhelms all other motives and that compels abstinent alcoholics to resume drinking.

The search to establish physical tolerance and withdrawal as the decisive cause of chronic heavy drinking has been abandoned by almost all researchers. There is evidence that, like genetic factors, these physical factors may play a role in influencing drinking behavior. But clearly many other factors must also come into play. After an extensive review of the data, one research team concluded that:

> The safest, indeed perhaps the only, thing that can be said is that under certain circumstances, tolerance and physical dependence may contribute to variation in [alcohol] consumption. . . . The question with which we are left is not really whether tolerance and physical dependence are important [in increasing the probability of drinking], but rather how they compare in importance to a host of other factors that also control alcohol consumption.[24]

At this point we need to clear up some popular misconceptions about the term *physical dependence*. Strictly speaking, physical dependence refers to the development of physical tolerance and withdrawal symptoms in a person who has used a particular substance over time. As we noted earlier, many long-term drinkers do develop a physical tolerance for alcohol and exhibit physical symptoms (tremors, anxiety, etc.) when they stop drinking.

But in everyday conversation, these physical developments are misinterpreted to mean that the substance abuser has an urgent need, an intense desire, a necessary reliance on the substance such that he "can't live without it." There is no scientific evidence whatsoever for this popular redefinition of *dependency*. In no known respect does a person who experiences the physical symptoms of alcohol dependence require—either subjectively or objectively—a drink of alcohol. Rather, abundant studies show that drinkers who suffer physical symptoms of withdrawal will often, and of their own volition, refrain from drinking.

It is true that drinkers who develop the symptoms of physical dependency are, other things being equal, more likely to continue drinking heavily than those who do not. The more severe the symptoms, the greater the likelihood of the drinker continuing to drink, and the lower the likelihood of returning to more moderate drinking. These general patterns have been documented in a four-year followup study of people admitted for inpatient alcohol treatment programs.[25] But while this study suggests general trends, the followup data do not illustrate any hard-and-fast relationships between physical dependency and subsequent drinking behavior. Of those drinkers who showed severe physical dependence symptoms at the time of admission, 12 percent were drinking without any physical symptoms or social problems at the four-year followup, and another 23 percent had been abstinent for at least a year. Among those who on admission had dependence symptoms at low levels, 30 percent were nonproblem drinkers four years later; another 20 percent had been abstinent for a year or more. And of those who on admission were abstinent or without dependence symptoms, about 31 percent were nonproblem drinkers at the followup, and about 16 percent had abstained for a year or more. Despite the statistically significant correlations between physical dependency and subsequent problem drinking, the substantial overlap in all categories indicates that physical dependency, whether severe or mild, is not a trustworthy predictor of how any individual drinker will behave.

A final point about this study raises an issue that always lurks in the background of efforts to relate physical dependency to subsequent behavior. As one might expect, the drinkers who had the stronger symptoms of dependency generally had been drinking much longer and more heavily than those who had mild symptoms or none at all. Thus the statistical correlations reported in this study may have far less to do with the effects of physical dependency than with the simple proposition that people who have been drinking heavily for a long time are likely to have more difficulty in changing their drinking behavior. Habits, associations, and life circumstances would mitigate against the probability of radical change, all quite independently of any physical symptoms. Rather than being a *cause* of heavy drinking, the physical symptoms may be just one more *consequence* of it.

## Psychological Hypotheses

Numerous attempts have been made to explain the alcoholic's patterns of drinking by reference to psychological constructs: personality, inner conflict, anxiety, poor self-image, and so on. We need not review all these theories, none of which has been scientifically confirmed and none of which has earned general acceptance in the scientific community.[26] Most are highly speculative, often based on studies of limited samples or clinical interpretations of individual cases.

In the late 1960s and early 1970s there was speculation that men drink heavily in order to hide self-perceptions of weakness, that their drinking represents a reaction against feelings of psychological dependency on others.[27] Other studies suggested that certain personality traits are statistically associated with a higher risk of becoming an alcoholic. But the sorts of traits in question are so broadly defined and are so common among nonalcoholics as well—impulsivity, dependency, inadequate self-esteem—as to be of little practical use. As one reviewer succinctly put it: "Studies of the personality of alcoholics have consistently led to a rejection of an 'alcoholic personality.'"[28]

Several psychosocial studies have, however, provided us with important statistical data on groups likely to be at risk for becoming alcohol abusers. Children of alcoholics are at higher risk in our society: Due to genetic and environmental factors, between 20 percent and 25 percent of males who have an alcoholic parent become alcoholics.[29] The other side of the coin: this finding equally implies that 75 percent to 80 percent of individuals in this high-risk group do not become alcoholics, and that most alcoholics do not have alcoholic parents. So, while this at-risk correlation is statistically significant in predicting national rates of alcoholism, it is useless as a predictor of any individual's destiny, since 75 percent to 80 percent of the time the "prediction" is not fulfilled.

Of equal importance: Even if in some cases genetic factors play a contributing role, whether the child of an alcoholic grows up to become a heavy drinker depends largely on the individual's social environment and life history.

Perhaps the most widely appealing types of psychological hypotheses are those proposing to explain long-term heavy drinking in terms of learning theory. The general premise of this approach is that people persistently drink heavily because they have "learned" to handle certain of life's challenges in this way. We have already discussed, and rejected, an operant conditioning hypothesis. Other applications of learning theory to alcohol abuse emphasize more complex phenomena such as cognition, emotion, and desire.

Although the key behaviors associated with long-term heavy drinking have never been accounted for in rigorous and quantifiable terms derived from learning theory, the jargon of learning theory is loosely adopted in some quarters. One may read of responses, reinforcements, and operant rewards, of learning schedules, cognitive-symbolic correlates, cognitive dissonance, personal attribution effects, and efficacy expectations. Sometimes these terms are used in a reasonably precise way to provide a context for an experiment or a theory. Often they are merely used as professional clichés for describing how people trying to cope with difficult situations adopt and give up various kinds of activities and over time develop preferred and even habitual ways of acting.

Whatever the ultimate adequacy of these theories, we realize that we have left the realm of medicine, disease, and physiological abnormality. All the explanations of alcoholism in terms of learning theory presume that the drinker's basic capacities for learning and unlearning are normal. The "abnormality" consists of the particular things they have learned to do—to repeatedly engage in conduct that has harmful or antisocial consequences—not of any impairment in their mental or physical learning capacities. In this context, *therapy* and *treatment* are medical-looking words that in substance refer to nonmedical procedures: to teaching heavy drinkers to do things other than drinking, and to have them learn to want to avoid heavy drinking.

While some drinkers may be helped by this approach, it is worth noting that we do not have a science of how to teach imprudent people to change and live prudently. And if learning theory should prove to provide a valid explanation for chronic alcohol abuse, then the medical issues of disease and cure, of psychological pathology, will be beside the point.

## Society and Culture

It is well established that all the manifold forms and patterns of heavy drinking are substantially affected by social, cultural, economic, and political factors.[30] The more one reads about the very different patterns of heavy drinking in various eras and cultures, the less plausible does it become that there is any one disease—one set of symptoms (a syndrome) uniquely associated with alcohol and its metabolism in the body—that could be the sole causal origin of chronic drinking.[31]

We know, for example, that all drinking patterns, including chronic heavy drinking, reflect cultural and ethnic norms. Relatively high proportions of the Irish, Scandinavian, and Russian populations (especially the adult males) drink a lot with some frequency. The French tradition, in contrast, has been one of drinking modest amounts at any one time but drinking frequently throughout the day, always remaining somewhat under the influence but rarely becoming visibly drunk, and eventually showing such physical signs as withdrawal. All sorts of cultural and subcultural norms, as well as such categories as geography and climate, socioeconomic class, and degree of urbanization have been significantly related to differences in drinking patterns.

Some cultures were first introduced to alcohol by the European explorers and colonists. Others had traditional ritual patterns of drinking and getting drunk that differed markedly from European behavior. For example, among the Chichicastenango Indians of Guatemala, there are two very different ways of drinking heavily. When drinking ceremonially, in the traditional way, men retain their dignity and fulfill their ceremonial duties even if they have drunk so much that they cannot walk unassisted. But when drinking in bars and taverns, where secular and European values and culture hold sway, the men dance, weep, quarrel, and act promiscuously.[32]

Similarly, in America today, we have different patterns for drinking at a formal dinner, at an informal meal in a private home, at a party, at a wedding, in a bar, with a group, and when alone. Social setting influences heavy drinkers as well. For example, one trained observer remarks that, in his experience, "astonishingly few alcoholics drink during their stay in hospital, despite having ample opportunities to do so. Yet an equally astonishing number of treated alcoholics return to drinking within a brief period of discharge."[33]

Another factor not commonly appreciated is economic: Under certain circumstances an increase in the cost of alcohol exerts a downward influence on the amount of drinking, including heavy drinking.[34] The evidence that even chronic heavy drinkers respond to the price of alcohol is that as prices increase, mortality from liver cirrhosis declines. (This is a useful indicator because liver cirrhosis occurs primarily among very heavy, very long-term drinkers, but it is quickly arrested if drinking stops.) We will return to the subject of pricing in Chapter 7, when we look at matters of public policy.

Another point to be mentioned here and elaborated upon in Chapter 7 is that political conditions can substantially affect heavy drinking. For example, rates of liver cirrhosis dropped dramatically in France during World War II and in the United States during Prohibition, and heavy drinking rose dramatically in Sweden when more liberal liquor-sale laws were adopted.[35]

## Conclusions

Research to date has shown that no one causal formula explains why people become heavy drinkers. Indeed, the attempt to find a single catchall "cause" of a single "disease" has repeatedly led researchers astray. On the basis of all the available evidence, many scientists are challenging *any* theory that assumes "[a] sharp distinction between the determinants of ordinary drinking and harmful drinking."[36]

There are, in short, many kinds of heavy drinking that arise from many different causes and produce many different patterns of associated problems. This recognition, after all these years of research, is not evidence of failure. It is an important and productive discovery, for we now know that we can give up the search for an explanation of a disease that does not exist. We can then look at the realities of alcohol abuse in our society and begin to think constructively about the variety of people and problems associated with alcohol abuse. As one researcher wrote recently, "The greatest advantage of the multivariate perspective is that it complicates the picture of alcohol-related difficulties and in so doing paints a picture that is credible and relevant to the needs of the individual case."[37] Instead of looking at heavy drinkers as victims of some wayward gene or physical abnormality, we can now see them in a truer light: as a diverse group of people who for diverse reasons are caught up in a particularly destructive way of life. Although this depiction is messier than any single-factor theory, it has the advantage of being true to the observations of clinicians, and to those of many heavy drinkers and their families and friends. Moreover, once alcohol abusers themselves realize that they have not been stricken by some unidentifiable physical or psychiatric condition, they may find new cause for hope and for a more realistic self-understanding.

## Notes

1. Edwards et al., *Alcohol and Alcoholism* (1979), 22–23. For a sense of the scientific consensus on single-factor models of causation, see Mello and Mendelson, *Alcohol: Use and Abuse in America* (1985), 230; Fingarette, "Philosophical and Legal Aspects of the Disease Concept of Alcoholism" (1983), 11; *Alcohol and Alcoholism* (1979), 89; Armor, Polich, and Stambul, *Alcoholism and Treatment* (1976), chap. 2; National Council on Alcoholism, "Criteria for the Diagnosis of Alcoholism" (1972); American Medical Association, *Manual on Alcoholism* (1967), 11.

2. Rohan, "Comments on the NCA Criteria Study" (1978), 211. On inconsistencies in the uses of *alcoholism* and *alcoholic*, see Mendelson and Mello, *The Diagnosis and Treatment of Alcoholism* (1985), 6; Fingarette (1983), 5–6; *Alcohol and Alcoholism* (1979), 10; Glatt, "Alcoholism Disease Concept and Loss of Control Revisited" (1976); Clark, "Conceptions of Alcoholism" (1975); Hore, *Alcohol Dependence* (1976), 44.

3. Jellinek, *The Disease Concept of Alcoholism* (1960), 12. On the use of the term *disease* in relation to alcoholism, see Fingarette (1983), 2–5; Fingarette and Hasse, *Mental Disabilities and Criminal Responsibility* (1979), 144–47; Fingarette, "The Perils of Powell" (1970), 808–12.

4. Saxe, Dougherty, and Esty, "The Effectiveness and Cost of Alcoholism Treatment" (1985), 489.

5. *Alcohol and Health* (1971), 71.

6. Cited in Maisto, Galizio, and Carey, "Individual Differences in Substance Abuse" (1985), 7.

7. For reviews, see Goodwin, "Genetic Determinants of Alcoholism" (1985); Deitrich and Spuhler, "Genetics of Alcoholism and Alcohol Actions" (1984).

8. Partanen, Bruun, and Markham, *Inheritance of Drinking Behavior* (1966); Kaij, *Alcoholism in Twins* (1960).

9. Goodwin et al., "Alcohol Problems in Adoptees Raised Apart from Alcoholic Biological Parents" (1973). Other relevant studies include Cloninger, Bohman, and Sigvardsson, "Inheritance of Alcohol Abuse" (1981); Cadoret and Gath, "Inheritance of Alcoholism in Adoptees" (1978); Schuckit, Goodwin, and Winokur, "A Study of Alcoholism in Half Siblings" (1972).

10. Cloninger, Bohman, and Sigvardsson (1981); Bohman, Sigvardsson, and Cloninger, "Maternal Inheritance of Alcohol Abuse" (1981); Cadoret and Gath (1978); Schuckit, Goodwin, and Winokur (1972).

11. Edwards et al. (1979), 108.

12. Survey data reported by Cahalan and Room, *Problem Drinking Among American Men* (1974), 28 and 74 (table 13).

13. An important line of thought, often labeled "constructivism," proposes an alternative concept of "the problem of alcohol" as a supposed major source of social troubles. As Joseph R. Gusfield has shown, the "problem of alcohol" is a social and symbolic construct that reflects social values and ideologies. For example, automobile accidents that involve a driver who has alcohol in his bloodstream are often perceived as alcohol-*caused* accidents even when faulty equipment, bad weather, or poor street design may have played a much larger role in causing the accident than the alcohol did. In spite of this, we construe the issue as an alcohol problem rather than a highway safety problem. See Gusfield, *The Culture of Public Problems* (1981) and *Symbolic Crusade* (1963); Wiener, *The Politics of Alcoholism* (1981); Levine, "The Discovery of Addiction" (1978); MacAndrew and Edgerton, *Drunken Comportment* (1969); Rudy, *Becoming Alcoholic* (1986).

14. Schuckit, *Drug and Alcohol Abuse* (1984), 61; Schuckit and Via-montes, "Ethanol Ingestion" (1979); Lindros, "Acetaldehyde—Its Metabolism and Role in the Action of Alcohol" (1978).

15. Lindros (1978), 159.

16. Schuckit (1984), 61.

17. Ludwig, Wikler, and Stark, "The First Drink" (1974).

18. Polich, Armor, and Braiker, *The Course of Alcoholism* (1980), 39 (table 3.10). See also Fingarette (1983), 7.

19. Mello, "A Semantic Aspect of Alcoholism" (1975), 83; Mello and Mendelson, "Drinking Patterns During Work-contingent and Non-contingent Alcohol Acquisition" (1972), 158.

20. Schuckit, "Charting What Has Changed" (1980), 71. For clinical observations, see Mendelson, "Experimentally Induced Chronic Intoxication and Withdrawal in Alcoholics" (1964), 119. For a summary of the inconsistencies between the positive reinforcement hypothesis and clinical data, see Mendelson and Mello, "One Unanswered Question about Alcoholism" (1979).

21. Pattison, Sobell, and Sobell, *Emerging Concepts of Alcohol Dependence* (1977), 101; Mendelson (1964), 119 and 122.

22. Mendelson and Mello (1979), 11.

23. Kissin, "The Disease Concept of Alcoholism" (1983), 109.

24. Cappell and LeBlanc, "Tolerance and Physical Dependence" (1981), 191. More recently, Tucker, Vuchinich, and Harris, "Determinants of Substance Abuse Relapse" (1985), 408, conclude that the literature shows the influence to be "minor," but some controversy persists on this point. In addition to Kissin (1983), see, for example, Edwards, "The Alcohol Dependence Syndrome" (1976). Edwards takes physical dependence to be a major causal factor, though not in itself decisive, in alcoholism. This hypothesis, however, lacks scientifically accepted proof.

25. Polich, Armor, and Braiker (1980), 59–62.

26. Vaillant and Milofsky's major, influential study concludes: "the etiological hypotheses that view alcoholism primarily as a symptom of psychological instability may be illusions"; "The Etiology of Alcoholism" (1982), 494. See also Mello and Mendelson (1985), 237. Here again, however, controversy continues; see Zucker and Gomberg, "Etiology of Alcoholism Reconsidered" (1986). For a review sympathetic to psychological approaches, see Cox, "Personality Correlates of Substance Abuse" (1985).

27. McClelland et al., *The Drinking Man* (1972); Blane, *The Personality of the Alcoholic* (1968).

28. Tarter, "Etiology of Alcoholism" (1978), 57. See also Polich, Armor, and Braiker (1980), 89–90; Orford and Edwards, *Alcoholism—A Comparison of Treatment and Advice* (1977), 119–20.

29. Goodwin (1985), 82–83.

30. A classic account in terms of the social context is MacAndrew and Edgerton (1969); for a concise review of the literature on cultural and ethnic norms, see Moser, *Prevention of Alcohol-Related Problems* (1980). See also Cahalan, "Subcultural Differences in Drinking Behavior" (1978), 245; Room, "Measurement and Distribution of Drinking Patterns and Problems in General Populations" (1977), 70–72.

31. See, for example, Holden, "Is Alcoholism Treatment Effective?" (1987), 20.

32. Marshall, "'Four Hundred Rabbits'" (1981), 192. For another ethnographical example, from among many, see Hill, "Alcohol Use Among the Nebraska Winnebago" (1987).

33. Heather and Robertson (1981), 143–44, referring to F. M. Canter, "The Requirement of Abstinence as a Problem in Institutional Treatment of Alcoholics" (1968).

34. P. Cook, "Increasing the Federal Alcohol Excise Tax" (1984).

35. Lenke, "Total Consumption of Alcohol and 'Heavy Use'" (1984).

36. Edwards et al. (1979), 23–24.

37. Caddy and Block, "Individual Differences in Response to Treatment" (1985), 354. For a full review, see Caddy, "Towards a Multivariate Analysis of Alcohol Abuse" (1978).

# CHAPTER 4

# Have "Alcoholism Treatments" Really Worked?

"Alcoholism is a disease, and alcoholism is treatable." That's the message conspicuously promoted by traditional alcoholism treatment programs* in their newspaper ads and TV commercials, on billboards and placards. This slogan is reinforced by the heartfelt testimonials of celebrities—politicians, writers, entertainers, sports figures—who write books and appear on talk shows to praise their newfound sobriety and thank the treatment program that showed them how to cope with their disease.

We have already seen that there is no scientific foundation for the first part of the slogan. No scientific research team has ever identified a biological cause that makes people become chronic heavy drinkers.

---

* In this chapter I use *traditional alcoholism treatment programs* to refer to a variety of programs based on variants of the classic disease concept. The criticisms made in this chapter refer only to those disease-oriented programs, not to the newer programs described in Chapter 6.

Nonetheless, the war on the supposed disease of alcoholism continues. The public hears a lot about newly opened treatment facilities; public support for government funding of treatment is strong; more drinkers are seeking treatment; and hospitals and private centers are doing a healthy business. Last year some 1.5 million Americans were seen in inpatient and outpatient treatment programs, with the bulk of their bill, about $1 billion, paid for by private health insurers.[1] And a stunningly broad diversity of alcoholism treatment programs are available: short-term and long-term programs; inpatient, outpatient, and mixed-setting programs; programs that focus on the drinker and the drinking itself, others that work with families and couples. Individual psychotherapy, group psychotherapy, confrontational tactics, dietary regimens, drugs, chemical aversion, biofeedback, relaxation training, behavioral conditioning, rational-emotive techniques, re-education, indoctrination, and self-help groups—all these methods and others are called into action.

What are we to make of this booming health-care industry that promises to treat a nonexistent disease? Could these programs be effective or worthwhile despite their faulty premise—that is, could they be doing the "right thing" for the "wrong reason"? Or are some or all of these programs playing on people's fears, spreading misinformation, and administering treatments that are no better than placebos?

For example, what are we to think of treatment programs whose advertisements compound myths, popular misconceptions, and untruths? Here's an excerpt from a typical ad—three sentences that promulgate three falsehoods:

> Willpower and strength of character have nothing to do with overcoming alcoholism.
> It is a complex disease that sends five out of six sufferers undiagnosed and unhelped to the grave.
> Call us today . . . because a drinking or drug problem rarely gets better by itself.

A persuasive piece of copywriting perhaps, but the consensus of scientific researchers is that willpower and personal strengths do affect the course of a heavy drinker's efforts to control his drinking: "Over and over we were impressed with the dominant role the patient, as opposed to the kind of treatment used on him, played both in his persistence in treatment and his eventual outcome."[2]

Furthermore, about one third of all heavy drinkers, including those diagnosed as alcoholics, improve over time without any treatment. This "maturing out" rate is even higher among drinkers who belong to the higher socioeconomic classes and those who have relatively stable personal and social lives.[3]

Certainly, instilling fear is a time-honored technique in advertising. But in the ad cited here we have a web of untruths. No wonder the author of an editorial in the *Journal of the American Medical Association* chastised the "competitive hype" and "carnival-like atmosphere" of the current ad wars.[4]

Yet the issues are far broader than bad faith in advertising. Are individual drinkers and their families being helped or hurt? Are public health-care funds and private medical insurance dollars being misspent on useless programs? Does the proliferation of treatment programs give us a false sense of security and distract our attention from our society's widespread problems with alcohol misuse and abuse?

"Alcoholism is treatable," the advertisements tell us. But what does this medical-sounding claim mean? Since the classic disease concept posits alcoholism as an incurable disease, "treatable" means that the adverse symptoms of the disease will be significantly eased or eliminated if the drinker undergoes certain recommended procedures and follows a specific followup regimen.

Moreover, the implication of "treatable" is that there is a scientifically proven cause-and-effect relationship between the therapeutic procedures and the subsequent course of the symptoms—in other words, that the treatment directly causes an improvement. But what if the improvement were to occur independent of the recommended treatment program? What if there was as much improvement after an hour or so of sensible professional advice as from an intensive inpatient program?

The current consensus in the research community is that by scientific standards of effectiveness the therapeutic claims of disease-oriented treatment programs are unfounded. The evidence is cumulative and consistent: None of these programs has ever been demonstrated to achieve improvement superior to any other type of help. Indeed, it has not been clearly demonstrated that such programs add anything at all to the improvement that could be expected in the natural course of affairs without a drinker's having received any professional help whatsoever. The very label *treatment* thus seems a deceptive misnomer. Before turning to the relevant studies of specific treatment regimens, I want to raise some general issues about the methods and goals of treatment programs based on the disease concept.

## Incoherent Doctrine and Practice

The aim of treatment programs based on the classic disease concept is to bring the alcoholic to a complete, permanent abstinence from alcohol. Abstention must be complete and permanent because, as the programs' literature emphasizes, the disease is incurable. That is to say, even after successful treatment the alcoholic is presumed to still have the same disease condition as when the symptom of uncontrolled drinking was manifest. But through treatment the alcoholic learns to refuse all alcohol, thus assuring that the deadly symptom of uncontrolled drinking will never be triggered by a first drink.

Yet, one must then ask proponents of the disease theory to

explain why elaborate treatment programs are needed to enable or teach alcoholics to abstain from the first drink. Why, once sober, would an alcoholic take a drink? After all, people who are seriously allergic to some food need only to be informed of what triggers the allergic reaction in order to be motivated to avoid eating that food. Why do alcoholics need to learn how to refuse a serving of the substance that triggers the serious reaction of uncontrolled drinking? More puzzlingly, why do alcoholics repeatedly turn to the very substance that triggers a loss of control?

As we have seen, one response to this puzzle is the conjecture that the disease also causes a loss of control over the choice to take or not take the first drink. But this conjecture totally undermines a standard procedure of most disease-oriented treatment programs, which demand that the alcoholic voluntarily stop drinking as a condition of admission into the program. Here is a truly troubling paradox: If the alcoholic's ailment is a disease that causes an inability to abstain from drinking, how can a program insist on voluntary abstention as a condition for treatment? (And if alcoholics who enter these programs do voluntarily abstain—as in fact they generally do—then of what value is the notion of loss of control?)

As for the treatment itself, the medical terminology (*disease, symptom, treatment*) implies that a medical regimen is used to address an essentially medical problem. One would therefore expect that the medical profession would have primary authority and responsibility for the treatment of heavy drinking. And in labeling alcoholism a disease, the medical profession does lay claim to primary expertise and authority in helping alcoholics. Yet almost all alcoholism treatment programs based on the disease concept use methods that do not belong to or derive from medical science or training. Alcoholics, of course, often need medical treatment for the diseases of the organs and the circulatory, nervous, and digestive systems that heavy drinkers exhibit at much higher rates, age for age, group for group, than social drinkers.[5] But clearly such medical treatments address the consequences of chronic heavy drinking, not the causes or the repetitive drinking behavior itself.

These programs may call upon medical personnel and techniques during detoxification. Yet this short-term medical aid only relieves the immediate distress of acute withdrawal; it is not in any way a treatment for alcoholism. Furthermore, professional medical attention is usually not necessary during detoxification. Even for diagnosed alcoholics, most often non-medical aid—a restful setting and emotional support—is sufficient.[6] Sometimes outpatient nursing aid and a moderate sedative are called for, but in fewer than 15 percent of all cases of withdrawal distress is medical intervention required. And hospitalization is necessary only if the detoxifying drinker exhibits gross physical and mental disorders (seizures, psychotic episodes, delirium tremens).

Even in these cases, however, the medical aid is addressed to alleviating the specific symptoms that arise on the occasion of detoxification. None of this medical assistance is intended to treat alcoholism; that is, no aspect of the medical intervention attacks the pattern of heavy drinking itself nor the drinker's stubborn propensity to resume drinking after detoxification. The role of medical doctors in treating the effects or symptoms of heavy drinking should not lead one to think that the medical profession has some special expertise in treating chronic drinking behavior. The truth is that medicine has had little or nothing to contribute in this regard.

Here again, then, the disease concept of alcoholism inevitably yields incoherences in theory and practice. Although the word *treatment* sounds like a medical term and many programs include some medical components, these programs are not medically based approaches to the so-called disease they would treat. The language of disease and treatment thus does not accurately describe the procedures and regimens of these programs; rather such language seems intended to legitimate a fast-growing health-services industry and to attract money and clients to it.

Differences of opinion exist among research authorities, but the basic finding of diverse studies and reviews of the literature is that if traditional alcoholism treatment programs help at all, it is not because of any specific medical or non-medical regimen. Whatever value these treatment programs have is modest at best, and it seems to reside not in the programs' particular techniques but in whatever practical advice and personal support they may give.[7]

Thus, while each program touts its own methods, there is no scientific evidence that any one disease-oriented program is any more effective than another:

> There is little definitive evidence that any one treatment or treatment setting is better than any other. Furthermore, controlled studies have typically found few differences in outcome according to intensity or duration of treatment. . . . There is little evidence for the superiority of either inpatient or outpatient care.

> [A] review of other studies of continuous abstinence from alcohol following treatment shows that various types of treatment do not influence continuous abstinence rates, particularly when the subjects are assessed at 12 months after treatment.[8]

The sole encouraging observation in these studies is the suggestion that some programs may be more effective for certain groups of drinkers and that matching the drinker to the most suitable program may yield better results. We will return to this conjecture in Chapter 6, but here must note that were it to be found true, some of the present disease-oriented programs might be able to achieve better results, but they would have to fully abandon the classic concept of alcoholism as one disease that indiscriminately affects all its victims.

Of course, some drinkers do improve during the course of a disease-oriented program, just as some drinkers improve with no treatment. The issue is whether any of this improvement can be ascribed to the program itself. All the scientific evidence suggests that clients' improvement is not due to the treatment program nearly so much as to natural influences and background forces (socioeconomic status, social stability, motivation, family setting): "it seems likely that treatment may often be quite puny in its powers in comparison to the sum of these background forces."[9]

After an extensive study of the literature, the authors of a report sponsored by the U.S. Congress, Office of Technology Assessment were willing to affirm only that "The conclusions of many of these reviews is that treatment seems better than no treatment." Even this cautiously qualified statement appears overly confident compared to the report issued by Vaillant after a highly ambitious and elaborate eight-year clinical experiment (CASPAR). Vaillant candidly concluded that "there is compelling evidence that the results of our treatment were no better than the natural history of the disease."[10]

Nor could Vaillant find any evidence of any positive effect specifically due to treatment in five comparable clinical studies that he carefully reviewed. Pessimistic, too, was his analysis of the results of ten long-term followup studies covering a wide variety of treatment methods. Two years after treatment, Vaillant explains, about 20 percent of the drinkers were abstinent, 15 percent continued drinking but showed improvement, and 65 percent were still abusing alcohol. Because these proportions were the same for a comparable population of drinkers who did not enter any treatment program, the best that can be said, Vaillant concluded, is that these programs didn't make matters worse.

In the aggregate, then, the strongest scientifically based claims that can be made by disease-oriented treatment programs is that the staff try to be supportive and helpful and that doing something may perhaps be a bit more effective—or at least no worse—than doing nothing for chronic heavy drinkers seeking assistance in controlling their drinking behavior.

## A Dose of Advice

In the mid-1970s a team of researchers in Great Britain conducted a rigorously designed large-scale experiment to test the effectiveness of a treatment program that represented "the sort of care which might today be provided by most specialized alcoholism clinics in the Western world."[11]

The subjects were one hundred men who had been referred for alcohol problems to a leading British outpatient program, the Alcoholism Family Clinic of Maudsley Hospital in London. The receiving psychiatrist confirmed that each of the subjects met the following criteria: he was properly referred for alcohol problems, was aged 20 to 65 and married, did not have any progressive or painful physical disease or brain damage or psychotic illness, and lived within a reasonable distance of the clinic (to allow for clinic visits and follow-up home visits by social workers). A statistical randomization procedure was used to divide the subjects into two groups comparable in the severity of their drinking and their occupational status.

For subjects in one group (the "advice group"), the only formal therapeutic activity was one session between the drinker, his wife, and a psychiatrist. The psychiatrist told the couple that the husband was suffering from alcoholism and advised him to abstain from all drink. The psychiatrist also advised the husband to stay on his job (or return to it) and encouraged the couple to attempt to keep their marriage together. There was free-ranging discussion and advice about the personalities and particularities of the situation, but the couple was told that this one session was the only treatment the clinic would provide. They were told in sympathetic and constructive language that the "attainment of the stated goals lay in their own hands and could not be taken over by others."

Subjects in the second group (the "treatment group") were offered a year-long program that began with a counseling session, an introduction to Alcoholics Anonymous, and prescriptions for drugs that would make alcohol unpalatable and drugs that would alleviate withdrawal suffering. Each drinker then met with a psychiatrist to work out a continuing outpatient treatment program, while a social worker made a similar plan with the drinker's wife. The ongoing counseling was focused on practical problems in the areas of alcohol abuse, marital relations, and other social or personal difficulties. Drinkers who did not respond well were offered inpatient admission, with full access to the hospital's wide range of services.

Twelve months after the experiment began, both groups were assessed. No significant differences were found between the two groups. Furthermore, drinkers in the treatment group who stayed with it for the full period did not fare any better than those who dropped out. At the twelve-month point, only eleven of the one hundred drinkers had become abstainers. Another dozen or so still drank but in sufficient moderation to be considered "acceptable" by both husband and wife. Such rates of improvement are not significantly better than those shown in studies of the spontaneous or natural improvement of chronic drinkers not in treatment. Or, as Vaillant once ironically remarked: "The best that can be said for our exciting treatment is that we are certainly not interfering with the normal recovery process." [12]

Though the sophistication and elaborateness of the design and resources of this British experiment have made it a landmark project, a similar experiment with sixty alcoholics had been reported in 1969. The results were of the same kind: After one year there was no evident difference between drinkers who had received intensive treatment and those who had received minimal treatment and had been told that the patient, not the program, had to deal with the problem.

Such experiments suggest that anything more than an hour or two of commonsense advice from an authoritative person may be a waste of time, money, and resources.[13] But, as we noted earlier, it may be that these large-scale studies oversimplify matters. Perhaps the effectiveness of treatment for some drinkers is statistically canceled out by the treatment's lack of effectiveness for others. If one method is used for different sorts of people and problems, and that method produces benefits for some, setbacks for others, and little or no effect on still others, the overall statistical data would show a net zero effect. In other words, perhaps some programs would prove effective if only they were administered to the right drinkers.

## Factors That Bias
## Claims of Effectiveness

If the scientific evidence does not support the effectiveness of disease-oriented programs, how do some programs and studies arrive at their claims of impressive success rates? For example, one British study reported that about 60 percent of the alcoholics who completed hospital programs showed substantial improvement one year after finishing the program.[14] These results appear significantly better than anything that could be attributed to natural improvement, which would predict progress for roughly 30 percent of the group. Furthermore, drinkers who enter hospital programs tend to have more severe symptoms of physical dependence—a point that makes the success rate look even better.

But, as the authors of the report note, the drinkers in these hospital programs were usually selected to enter the special treatment regimens because they were considered well motivated for treatment and showed no severe personality, physical, or neurological disorders. Thus the most severe cases— drinkers who had developed deteriorating physical or mental conditions—were screened out. In the judgment of the report's authors, then, the inpatients were not typical; in effect, "the cards [were] stacked" to produce good results. Had the inpatients been a typical group, the authors estimate that favorable results would have dropped to about 20 percent to 30 percent—well within the range of natural improvement.

Another influential factor unrelated to the actual treatment regimen is the fact that many drinkers enter a treatment program precisely at a time when their drinking problems have become particularly acute. They finally come for help because they have reached a low point. In a sense, they have nowhere to go but up; on a purely statistical basis, their entry at a low point strongly increases the probability of a significant improvement on the average at a later followup.[15] Moreover anyone with the motivation to voluntarily endure the rigors of such an intensive inpatient program is, all else being equal, statistically more likely to show improvement than someone not as motivated.[16] Once having gone through the program, those who improve will ascribe their improvement to the ordeal endured and will tend to become ardent advocates for that particular method.

Another factor that biases claims about improvement rates is that programs typically publicize the rate of improvement for drinkers who complete the program. But the dropouts— often quite a few—are typically not included as failures. Nor do most programs follow up on their dropouts to see if any of them succeed despite having left the program. When long-term followup studies are conducted of program graduates, persons who have died of causes related to resumed drinking are often not counted among the graduates, and so their failure to control their drinking does not figure in the "survivor improvement rate."[17]

One recent study, for example, found that among 677 cases of alcoholics followed up two years after a hospital admission for alcoholism treatment, the death rate for those who continued to misuse alcohol was 60.4 per 1,000 persons, eight times greater than the 7.7 per 1,000 that would have been expected for nonabusers matched for age, sex, and race.[18] If the alcohol-abusing deceased and 46 non-traceable cases (some of whom may have been unfindable because of alcohol misuse or death from alcohol-related causes) were added to the failure rate, the hospital program's sucess rate would drop from the reported 46 percent to 30–35 percent, within the range of natural improvement.

If an alcoholism treatment program draws from well-educated, middle- or upper-class whites who are married, employed, and middle-aged or older, the reported success rates will look particularly good. Such persons have roughly twice the natural improvement rate of drinkers of low socio-economic status.[19] Since individuals with higher socioeconomic status and more socially stable lives tend to predominate among the patients in the more elaborate and expensive treatment programs, the success rates for such programs often look very good: many clients do improve. But the treatment per se will have had little or no measurable effect on the program's clients, the same number of whom would have predictably improved without treatment.

The key role of the personal characteristics of drinkers entering treatment is highlighted in studies of the Schick-Shadel program.* Early reports of high success rates for this program

---

* The cornerstone of the Schick-Shadel program is a form of conditioning by negative reinforcement: At intervals over a five-day period, the drinker is offered liquor to taste or smell while he is under the influence of a powerful nausea-inducing drug. The premise is that the drinker will thereafter as-

noted that almost all of the drinkers treated had paid substantial sums for the program, which implies that they were highly motivated and of at least moderate socioeconomic status. In contrast, "over a hundred charity cases [were] treated, but the result [was] discouraging." [20]

A sympathetic account of the high success rates for the Schick-Shadel and Raleigh Hills programs summarizes the issues this way:

> Why do these outcome data appear to be so much better than those from other approaches to alcoholism? One answer is that alcoholics undergoing chemical aversion treatment now, as in the 1940s, probably enter treatment with better prognoses than those who enter most other kinds of treatment. To begin with, patients entering chemical aversion programs (which are costly) must have substantial private financial resources or health insurance, both of which would require them to be either recently or still employed. Recent or current employment suggests a modicum of ability to function adequately in the world. Further, these patients also differ in educational and socioeconomic level from alcoholics treated elsewhere, additional indications of their superior treatment potential. Finally, patients who complete a chemical aversion treatment sequence must be highly motivated to change their drinking behavior because the treatment is both expensive and extremely unpleasant. It is well accepted, of course, that positive treatment motivation is one of the most important predictors of successful treatment. [21]

Distorted success rates also appear in studies that use short followup times. Especially if abstinence is the program goal, the rate of relapse rises significantly subsequent to the first six months after leaving the program. An eighteen-month followup seems a more reliable indicator of long-term results. [22]

Unfortunately, the accurate assessment of drinkers on admission to a program and the evaluation of success rates over long periods of time require elaborate experimental designs,

---

sociate the nausea with the liquor and his urge to drink will decline or disappear.

implementation, and followup.[23] The expertise and expense are beyond the resources of the typical treatment program. Moreover, program staff often do not have the expertise to appreciate the shortcomings of their program's informal self-evaluation nor the value of carefully conducted assessments that appear in the scientific literature. For even professional staff members are primarily treatment-oriented and are generally not trained or interested in research methodology. They may be expert practitioners, but nonetheless be quite naive about the conduct and evaluation of scientific research.

Thus the program staff may put their hearts and souls into their work and be genuinely convinced that they are achieving outstandingly successful results. And their genuine conviction persuades nonpractitioners. But research scientists insist on higher and more objective standards when evaluating the outcome of a treatment program. And their consensus is that any treatment can look good on paper but still lack validity: "Reflecting . . . spontaneous improvements or responses to informal and nonspecific interventions, any treatment can look good. The field is full of stories of new 'cures,' seemingly effective when offered as part of an uncontrolled investigation, only to be proven later to be no better than a placebo."[24]

Having examined some of the social, statistical, and experimental factors that influence and distort measures of a treatment's success rate, we can now look at a few specific treatment methods.

### Disulfiram (Antabuse)

One of the widely used methods of treatment for alcohol abuse is the administration of the chemical disulfiram, marketed under the trade name Antabuse. After a dosage of Antabuse, any ingestion of alcohol will cause nausea, vomiting, breathing difficulties, and profuse sweating. Indeed, the reaction is so strong that Antabuse must be prescribed with caution; it can produce lasting harm or even death if taken in sufficient doses by people who have heart conditions or certain other ailments.[25]

The use of Antabuse seems intuitively reasonable: the chemical effectively makes it impossible for anyone to drink any beverage with alcohol in it. Even the description of the violent reaction can be enough to frighten a patient from trying to take a drink.

But the success of Antabuse depends entirely on the drinker's willingness to consistently take the drug. That is, the chemical provides a prop for a drinker who is already, for other reasons, strongly enough committed to abstention to remain on a schedule of doses of Antabuse. If a drinker does not have a strong will to stop heavy drinking, he may resist a casual impulse to drink because of the Antabuse he has already ingested, but he could also skip several doses and then resume drinking. In a nutshell, Antabuse eliminates drinking, but the drinker can always decide to eliminate the Antabuse.

One careful study reported that a tiny, pharmacologically inactive dose of Antabuse produced abstinence rates as high as the full active dose.[26] This finding confirms the view that the belief one is taking Antabuse, and no doubt the fear of the effect, is as effective as taking the chemical itself. Drinkers in this study who attended the outpatient clinic more regularly—a voluntary activity—were more likely to continue the Antabuse and to remain abstinent; but drinkers who wanted to drink simply stopped taking the Antabuse for three or more days. Subjects who were employed were more likely to stay with the Antabuse and thus remain abstinent. So, once again, initial motivation and socioeconomic stability bear on the likelihood of the choice to remain abstinent.[27] This study, one of the most positive in the literature, concluded that any specific effect of the Antabuse was at best limited.

More generally, the reviews and summaries of the relevant scientific literature fail to support the method:

Although disulfiram has been used in treatment of alcoholism for almost 35 years, problems in designing an adequate experiment make it difficult to say just how useful it is. Controlled studies are few, and in those which have been carried out the difference between disulfiram and those given placebo are minimal.[28]

Similarly noncommittal results were reported in a recent large-scale study conducted in nine Veterans Administration hospitals around the nation.[29] Nevertheless, Antabuse continues to be widely and confidently used as a mainstay of alcoholism treatment.

## Psychopharmacology:
## Antidepressants and Tranquilizers

Antidepressants and tranquilizers are also used in alcoholism treatment programs, and a large number of private physicians who treat alcoholism prescribe drugs of some kind. Physicians who assume that depression underlies heavy drinking prescribe antidepressant drugs; those who assume some other psychiatric condition, perhaps neurotic anxiety or schizophrenic processes, prescribe one or another kind of tranquilizer.

As we have seen, however, there is no scientific evidence that heavy drinking is caused by a specific psychiatric condition. There is therefore no sound medical rationale to treat alcoholic patients generally with antidepressants or tranquilizers. Indeed, almost three-fourths of diagnosed alcoholics do not show significant signs of any psychiatric disorder; these drinkers are said to have "primary alcoholism."[30] For drinkers diagnosed as having "secondary alcoholism" (chronic heavy drinking specifically associated with an independently diagnosed mental disorder), drugs may be needed to treat the mental disorder, and alleviating that disorder may in turn favorably affect the drinking behavior. But in such cases, the persistent heavy drinking is not a symptom of a specific disease of alcoholism, but is instead a secondary effect of an independently treatable mental disorder.

In any case, the data do not substantiate any overall success of drug therapies of any kind in preventing or ameliorating heavy drinking. One review of eighty-nine studies of programs using drugs to treat alcoholism concluded that "no drug has been proven to be better than a placebo in the treatment of chronic alcoholics."[31] This reviewer also observed that 95 percent of the programs that did not use a control group claimed some success, but only 5 percent of the programs that did use a control group for comparison made the same claim. Here again, careful experimental design makes the difference. In the absence of a control group (a comparable group of subjects who do not receive the treatment but are monitored along with those subjects who do receive the treatment), any treatment program can claim success for drinkers whose recovery was due to natural improvement.

### Alcoholics Anonymous (A.A.)

A.A. seems to call for special comment because it is so widely recommended by professionals of all orientations, so fervently testimonialized by its members, and so prominent in the public mind. The A.A. model has also had enormous influence on the organization of self-help groups for relatives and children of alcoholics and for gamblers, overeaters, and others whose behavior seems to fit the "addictive" pattern.

A.A. groups provide individual members with powerful moral and emotional support, as well as practical aid and advice—provided the member conforms to the key expectations of the group. There are frequent meetings, with a strong confessional element. Members are encouraged to search their souls and their memories, and they are expected to gradually discover therein a personal history that by and large conforms to the A.A. picture of the course of alcoholism. Members whose memories or understanding of their experiences are inconsistent with A.A. doctrine may be confronted and charged with denial. The group exerts a powerful form of peer pressure on new members to see themselves and explain themselves in terms of the A.A. picture of an alcoholic.

Members who would fully participate must therefore acknowledge that they have an incurable progressive disease, which they are powerless as individuals to overcome. They must accept total abstention as their only hope. They must profess their reliance on a Higher Power and commit themselves to helping fellow members discover these truths and fight off drink. The emotional pitch and the sense of comradeship, in both despair and hope, can be intense. Not surprisingly, those who become regular A.A. members do learn to believe in an autobiography that exemplifies A.A. teaching and to gloss over or ignore experiences and feelings that are contradicted by the teaching.[32] For them, A.A. often becomes an alternative way of life, which is as intensely focused on abstinence as their former lives had been focused on alcohol. This passionate and complete reorientation is not a unique phenomenon; it is rather like what critics of sects would call ideological re-education or a modest form of elective brainwashing.

Despite the ubiquitous good opinion of A.A., there are no satisfactory data to justify the widespread confidence in it, in part because A.A. has long been reluctant to gather or publish statistics. The evidence of A.A.'s success is thus anecdotal, impressionistic, and suffused with sectarian fervor. But disinterested researchers have observed and studied the organization in efforts to evaluate its therapeutic claims.

A key factor in assessing A.A.'s efficacy is the program's highly self-selective nature. Estimates made in 1974 put A.A. membership in Canada and the U.S. at no more than about

5 percent of all alcoholics. While this small percentage represents a sizable number of people, as one researcher notes, it is "well known to everyone actively engaged in the field . . . [that] the A.A. programme of recovery is simply not acceptable or attractive to the majority of people suffering problems from drinking."[33]

As we have seen, selectivity in the kind of drinkers who enter a treatment regimen biases the outcomes and precludes any generalization about the regimen's success with heavy drinkers or problem drinkers at large. Drinkers who become active participants in A.A. are those who are willing to affirm themselves as alcoholics under the A.A. definition; drinkers who do not fit or will not acknowledge fitting the pattern drop out.

The public is often impressed by the argument that drinkers who do persist in A.A. remain abstinent. But a number of researchers lean toward the converse: Drinkers remain in A.A. only if they are able to remain reasonably abstinent and also accept the A.A. way of life. The vast majority of heavy drinkers never try A.A., and most who do join drop out.

For example, one large-scale study of alcoholics in treatment centers in the U.S. found that 71 percent of their subjects had attended A.A. at some point; but at eighteen-month and subsequent followups only 14 percent to 18 percent were attending.[34] Moreover, the rate of problems was higher for irregular A.A. attenders than for either regular attenders or nonattenders. Among those who were regular A.A. attenders at the time of the initial interview, only 22 percent consistently maintained abstention up through the thirty-month followup interview, and over 33 percent had not only returned to drinking but also showed alcohol-related physical symptoms and life problems. A review of the literature about "slipping" from abstinence concluded that among A.A. members "slipping is a normal and frequent activity."[35]

Vaillant, one of the leading researchers most sympathetic

to A.A., nevertheless acknowledges that "at present the actual effectiveness of A.A. has not been adequately assessed."[36] Perhaps as fair a summary as any of the relevant scientific literature was prepared by the U.S. Congress, Office of Technology Assessment:

> AA is regarded by some as the most effective form of treatment of alcoholism—more effective than any of the approaches that professionals offer. Various problems with specifying the population that uses AA and a lack of data make such conclusions regarding AA's effectiveness difficult to verify or discount. Baeklund (1977), in his review of literature about AA, reports a 34% success rate—much lower than some of the earlier figures.
>
> Other reviewers have reported abstinence rates from 45% to 75%, depending on the length of the reporting period (Leach and Norris, 1977). The problem in evaluating AA is that its members probably differ from the general population of alcoholics, but data supporting this statement as well as other data about AA are difficult to obtain (Baeklund, 1977). Although a substantial number of regular attendees are abstinent (AA, 1972), it is unclear how this relates to the number who try the program. Because nonabstainers may be subjected to ridicule and reproach by other members, it is probably more likely than not that those who remain in AA for long periods of time are those who have achieved sobriety. It seems clear that some aspects of AA programs have useful therapeutic roles (e.g., getting alcoholics to acknowledge their problem, providing a support system), but AA may only be applicable to some categories of alcoholics and alcohol abusers.[37]

It deserves note, as a final word on A.A., that while the group's doctrine holds that alcoholism is a disease, the practice of A.A. is entirely nonmedical. A.A. is not a treatment, but a new way of life for those who choose to become involved. Members join a community that fosters intense emotional bonds, provides an integrated set of values and priorities, with powerful symbols and rituals, and offers frequent social activities and an active network of communication. For regular members the A.A. campaign against alcohol comes to replace drinking as an activity central to their daily lives and identity.

This view of A.A. as essentially a new way of life, rather than as a treatment program, recalls remarks that Vaillant made after the failure of his elaborately designed treatment program. He wondered if what many heavy drinkers needed was to participate in an "emotionally charged but communally shared ritual, and a shared belief system," one that offered confidence, faith, and hope—although "hope is unscientific." [38] Not medicine, then, he suggests, but a new form of social organization and communication might lead heavy drinkers to a new way of life. In Part Two we will return to this theme of personal and social life patterns. But here we must note that there is no evidence that the particular way of life advocated by A.A. is the only, or even the most effective, application of this theme. The A.A. way of life is one way, but the proposition that alcoholism is one all-encompassing and selfsame disease to be defeated only by one all-healing alternative is a barrier to progress for most heavy drinkers.

## Conclusions

The claim that alcoholism is a treatable disease turns out to be fraught with ambiguity and vagueness, and there is no scientific evidence to support it. Among members of the treatment establishment, there may seem to be agreement on the highly generalized claim that alcoholism can be successfully treated. But if we press the inquiry, we find even as professional and paraprofessional treatment staff roundly agree that we now know how to treat alcoholism, adherents of competing programs routinely challenge one another's facts, findings, and conclusions. In the absence of any scientific evidence to support their claims, treatment staff and administrators fall back on partisan loyalty to their own programs.

Every year a certain proportion of heavy drinkers do moderate their drinking or choose abstinence for shorter or longer periods of time. But neither the rate nor the duration of this natural improvement is predictably affected by participation in a traditional alcoholism treatment program: "Many long-term studies of the course of alcoholism concur that treatment has little if any lasting effect." Or, in the words of another leading scientific researcher: "For all that has been said, written, and done about the treatment of alcohol problems, we still appear to be at the beginning of the beginning."[39]

That disease-oriented treatment programs have failed to prove their effectiveness is only part of the story, however. The very prevalence of the disease concept has had a range of adverse effects on all aspects of society's efforts to understand or help heavy drinkers. First, the disease concept focuses disproportionate resources on the small minority of heavy drinkers who are diagnosed as having the so-called disease, all the while providing heavy drinkers who do not fit the pattern of symptoms with a rationalization for denying that they have serious drinking problems.

Second, the disease concept mistakenly focuses attention on medical intervention as the key to treatment; evidence about the role of social, psychological, and other nonmedical factors is largely ignored. In turn, this medical approach reduces the drinking behavior of the chronic drinker to a physical symptom, thereby both encouraging the heavy drinker to evade responsibility for drinking and also encouraging the drinker and others to interpret the drinking as a reflexive symptom imposed by a disease, rather than to understand the drinking as a meaningful though maladaptive activity.

Finally, the disease concept poses a frustrating paradox for drinkers who do seek treatment: They are told that they are the unwilling victims of a disease that destroys their ability to manage their drinking and yet that they must strive to exert absolute self-control, that only total abstinence can save them.

# Notes

1. Saxe, Dougherty, and Esty, "The Effectiveness and Cost of Alcoholism Treatment" (1985), 488 and 516–18. See also Holden, "Alcoholism and the Medical Cost Crunch" (1987a), 1132; Holden, "Is Alcoholism Treatment Effective?" (1987b), 23; W. Miller and Hester, "Inpatient Alcoholism Treatment" (1986), 794.

2. Baeklund, Lundwall, and Kissin, "Methods for the Treatment of Chronic Alcoholism" (1975), 305. For a review of the main types of programs, see Saxe, Dougherty, and Esty (1985), 492–98; Marlatt, "Psychosocial Perspectives on Alcoholism and the Process of Recovery" (1982).

3. On natural improvement, see Vaillant, *The Natural History of Alcoholism* (1983), 284; Schuckit, "Alcoholism" (1977), 1814; Clare, "How Good Is Treatment?" (1976), 287. Brownell et al., "Understanding and Preventing Relapse" (1986), 766, conclude that "The vast majority of [addicted] persons who change do so on their own."

   On natural improvement in diagnosed alcoholics, see Tuchfield, "Spontaneous Remission in Alcoholics" (1981); Smart, "Spontaneous Recovery in Alcoholics" (1975). On the influences of socioeconomic class and stability of personal life, see Cahalan and Room, *Problem Drinking Among American Men* (1974), 51–52; Baeklund, Lundwall, and Kissin (1975), 271 and 305.

4. Tennant, "Disulfiram Will Reduce Medical Complications but Not Cure Alcoholism" (1986), 1489.

5. Mendelson et al., "Alcoholism and Prevalence of Medical and Psychiatric Disorders" (1986); Popham, Schmidt, and Israelstam, "Heavy Alcohol Consumption and Physical Health Problems" (1985); R. Moore, "The Prevalence of Alcoholism in Medical and Surgical Patients" (1985).

6. Schuckit, *Drug and Alcohol Abuse* (1984), 46; W. Miller and Hester (1986), 795.

7. Baeklund, Lundwall, and Kissin (1975), 307.

8. The two sources cited are Saxe et al., "The Effectiveness and Costs of Alcoholism Treatment" (1983), 4–5, and Tennant (1986), 1489. For another comparison of inpatient and outpatient treatment, see W. Miller and Hester (1986), 794.

9. Orford and Edwards, *Alcoholism—A Comparison of Treatments and Advice* (1977), 118.

10. The two sources quoted in this paragraph are Saxe et al. (1983), 53, and Vaillant (1983), 123.

11. Orford and Edwards (1977), 11. For the researchers' description of the experimental protocol summarized here, see pages 39–42; for their statement of their key findings, see pages 54–57.

12. Vaillant, "The Doctor's Dilemma" (1980), 18.

13. WHO Expert Committee on Problems Related to Alcohol Consumption, *Problems Related to Alcohol Consumption* (1980), 46.

14. Study reported and assessed by Edwards et al., *Alcohol and Alcoholism* (1979), 130–31.

15. Polich, Armor, and Braiker, *The Course of Alcoholism* (1980), 82. See also Vaillant, "The Contribution of Prospective Studies in the Understanding of Etiologic Factors in Alcoholism" (1984), 281.

16. Nathan and Niaura, "Behavioral Assessment and Treatment of Alcoholism" (1985), 423. Orford, "Alcoholism" (1976), 92–93.

17. On the two biases mentioned in this paragraph, see Polich, Armor, and Braiker (1980), 176 and 98.

18. Barr et al., "Mortality of Treated Alcoholics and Drug Addicts" (1984). See also L. Sobell and M. Sobell, "Alcohol Treatment Outcome Evaluation Methodology" (1982), 303.

19. Baeklund, Lundwall, and Kissin (1975), 271 and 305. See also Saxe, Dougherty, and Esty (1985), 490; Costello, "Alcoholism Treatment Effectiveness" (1980); Polich, Armor, and Braiker (1980), 111.

20. Cited in Hore, *Alcohol Dependence* (1976), 123.

21. Nathan and Niaura (1985), 423. Frawley, "Neurobehavioral Model of Addiction" (1987) presents an elaborate model of the Schick-Shadel method but does not provide any evidence of its validity.

22. L. Sobell and M. Sobel (1982), 304; Polich, Armor, and Braiker (1980), 63–66.

23. See, for example, LaPorte et al., "Treatment Outcome as a Function of Follow-up Difficulty in Substance Abusers" (1981).

24. Schuckit (1977), 1814.

25. Jaffe and Ciraulo, "Drugs Used in the Treatment of Alcoholism" (1985), 369: "One recent large-scale study had to exclude about 17% of a total population of alcoholics in treatment because their medical condition contraindicated prescribing of Antabuse"; the

study referred to is Fuller et al., "Disulfiram Treatment of Alcoholism" (1986). See also Tennant (1986).

26. Fuller and Roth, "Disulfiram for the Treatment of Alcoholism"
(1979). See also Fuller and Williford, "Life-table Analysis of Abstinence in a Study Evaluating the Efficacy of Disulfiram" (1980).

27. See also Saxe et al. (1983), 52.

28. Jaffe and Ciraulo (1985), 369–70. See also Schuckit, "A One-Year
Follow-up of Men Alcoholics Given Disulfiram" (1985a), 191–95;
Fuller and Williford (1980); Fuller and Roth (1979).

29. Fuller et al. (1986), 1449.

30. Schuckit, *Drug and Alcohol Abuse* (1984), 48.

31. Viamontes, "Review of Drug Effectiveness in the Treatment of
Alcoholism" (1972), 1571. See also Schuckit (1977), 1814.

32. Shaw et al., *Responding to Drinking Problems* (1978), 58; see also
Keller, "On the Loss-of-Control Phenomenon in Alcoholism"
(1972). Edwards et al., "Alcoholics Anonymous" (1967) discuss
how the A.A. picture becomes a self-fulfilling prophecy. For
fuller, more sympathetic accounts see Robinson, *Talking Out of
Alcoholism* (1979), and Rudy, *Becoming Alcoholic* (1986).

33. Estimates of membership and quoted comment from Shaw et al.
(1978), 108 and 109.

34. Polich, Armor, and Braiker (1980), 126–30.

35. Rudy (1986), 71.

36. Vaillant (1983), 198.

37. Saxe, Dougherty, and Esty (1985), 514. The three sources cited in
this passage are: F. Baeklund, "Evaluation of Treatment Meth-
ods in Chronic Alcoholism," in B. Kissin and H. Begleiter, eds.,
*Treatment and Rehabilitation of the Chronic Alcoholic* (New York:
Plenum Press, 1977); B. Leach and F. L. Norris, "Factors in the
Development of Alcoholics Anonymous (A.A.)," in the same
volume; Alcoholics Anonymous, *Profile of an AA Meeting* (New
York: Alcoholics Anonymous World Service, 1972).

38. Vaillant (1983), 288 and 291.

39. The two sources quoted in this paragraph are Vaillant (1983),
147, and Glaser, "Anybody Got a Match?" (1980), 193.

PART 2

---

# New Approaches
# to Heavy Drinking

CHAPTER 5

---

# Understanding Heavy Drinking as a Way of Life

Once we free ourselves of the discredited classic disease concept, we no longer limit our attention to a relatively small group of diagnosed alcoholics whose drinking behavior allegedly derives from a single causal origin and follows a single inexorable course. Instead we perceive a much larger and more diverse assortment of individual heavy drinkers who have little in common except that (1) they drink a lot, (2) they tend to have many more problems in life than nondrinkers or moderate drinkers, and (3) they show a puzzlingly inconsistent ability to manage their drinking.

As researchers continue to put together all the scientific evidence, scientists have come to see that no one explanation of alcohol dependence can account for all the behavior of all these drinkers. As one reviewer puts it, "The search for the 'magic bullet' has given way to the recognition that the disorder is as complex as the person who suffers it."[1]

The broad interpretation that best fits the evidence is that heavy drinkers are people for whom drinking has become a central activity in their way of life. By "central activity" I mean any hub of activity (job, religious practice, serious hobby, family or community role) that in part defines and inspires a person's identity, values, conduct, and life choices. For example, in some people's lives religion is a central activity, a main thread around which life is woven, while for others religion is merely a traditional Sunday churchgoing routine, an incidental decoration, as it were. For some people food or gambling are valued pleasures and recreational activities, but their role is circumscribed; whereas for others life comes to revolve around food or around gambling. Just so, for some people having a drink or two is a pleasant occasional practice, but for the long-term heavy drinker life has come to center on drinking—life is pervaded by a preoccupation with drinking, shaped and driven by the quest for drink, drinking situations, and drinking friends.

Central activities exert far more power on our conduct and have far stronger implications for behavior than one might assume. In order to clarify this power and influence, I will at each point in the following discussion offer an example of a central activity that does not concern alcohol before applying the insight to heavy drinking.

## Central Activities
## and Ways of Life

Each of us has developed a particular way of life. For most of us, our way of life is not all of a simple, neat, coherent piece—there are loose ends, worn spots, and some weakly patched-together seams. The warp and woof of one's way of life are the various activities that one engages in and one's individual way of performing these activities.

For example, I am a university professor and devote a good portion of my time to teaching, talking to students, reading, and writing. My professional roles and responsibilities are outlined for me by my university and yet I fulfill them in my own style, at my own pace and rhythm, and according to my own values and attitudes. And just as my professorial activities affect and color much of the rest of my life, so too do my other central activities color my professional conduct. My family life and my professional life continuously inform and influence one another.

To say heavy drinking is a *central activity* for someone is to say that it is an activity of the same order for that person as my vocation is for me. Our central activities tell something about what we each do with a meaningful portion of our time. Yet far more is at stake than the appropriation of time. For a central activity affects the style and nature of all aspects of our lives and interacts with all our other central activities.

Let's take reading as an example. For people who consider themselves avid readers, reading is a focal activity that occupies much of their thinking and conversation, that plays a role in their choice of friends and occupation. Even the furnishing of the reader's home will reflect the importance of this central activity: chairs and reading lights, bookshelf-lined walls, tables stacked with magazines. Similarly, a person's central activities exclude certain types of phenomena. Avid readers tend to avoid ways of life that leave no time for reading, just as nonreaders tend to avoid bookish settings, bookish people, and bookish occupations. Thus, in an important sense, though each of us initially makes choices that eventually determine our central activities, once an activity becomes central it influences, inspires, or even seems to demand certain other choices that further define who we are, how we act, where we go, and what we value.

In an analogous way, as heavy drinking becomes a central activity in the drinker's life, it shapes his or her daily schedule, friendships, domestic life, and occupational choices. Heavy drinkers tend to organize their lives to minimize contact with people who frown on drinking or condemn excessive drinking. And they tend to seek out people and situations that evoke and stimulate drinking—choices reinforced by various socially acceptable settings, rituals, and justifications for drinking.

Now, one may ask how a person comes to choose certain central activities but not others. Among my faculty colleagues and their career choices, no one answer holds. One of my colleagues took an academic career for granted because his parents were both professors; another was the child of immigrants who wanted professional careers for their children as a sign of having "arrived"; a third was captivated by a certain field of study and found that she had the talents to match her interests; a fourth sought the academic life as a form of retreat from the workaday world. These core motives were, of course, influenced by a host of other factors: a particularly inspiring professor who served as one's mentor, an appreciation of the high social status generally conferred on academics, the availability of fellowships and teaching posts, the encouragement of friends, and so on.

If we now look at heavy drinkers in the same light, our answer to the question of why some people become heavy drinkers is that there is no one general answer. Heavy drinkers are people who have over time made a long and complex series of decisions, judgments, and choices of commission and omission that have coalesced into a central activity.

But why, one asks, would someone make decisions that lead to a way of life so self-destructive and so injurious to others? The same sort of question can be asked in one respect or another of most of us. Why do we come to live in ways that are imprudent, harmful, or self-defeating? (And who does not do so in at least some aspect of life?) Why does someone repeatedly overspend and continually borrow ever greater sums in order to cover debts coming due? One choice, one act leads to another. We do not foresee, we do not intend the long-term pattern, but a series of individual quick-fix solutions may lead us into one.

These are profoundly important matters for each of us, but there is no one reason that motivates all our self-defeating conduct. The general truth is this: Human beings do not always respond wisely and with foresight; we often drift, unwitting, into a tangled web of decisions, expectations, habits, tastes, fears, and dreams. The chronic heavy drinker is no exception—no more mysterious, no less vulnerable. For the person challenged by personal problems, heavy drinking is one of the culturally available responses, however imprudent and self-destructive.

Thus, instead of positing an invisible breakdown in the machinery of self-control, we must start to look at heavy drinkers as people who are living—sometimes obliviously, sometimes quite consciously and painfully—with the consequences and ramifications of one of their central activities. Instead of viewing heavy drinkers as the helpless victims of a disease, we come to see their drinking as a meaningful, however destructive, part of their struggle to live their lives. This approach will enable us to better understand the heavy drinker's difficulties in acknowledging there is a drinking problem, or in making a resolution to control the drinking, or in abiding by that resolution.

## The Momentum of Central Activities

We have briefly illustrated some of the ways in which central activities intersect and contribute to one's total way of life. An even more profound phenomenon is how our way of life influences our perceptions of the world. For example, suppose there are three people approaching a downtown building: a real estate investor, an architecture buff, and a patient arriving for minor surgery at a doctor's office. Each of the three perceives the building in an entirely different way. The investor sees a piece of property in an up-and-coming neighborhood that represents a good business opportunity; the architecture buff pauses to appreciate a fine example of Louis Sullivan's influence on early-twentieth-century skyscrapers; the anxious patient may barely notice anything but the clock near the elevators.

At times, like the nervous patient, we find that our responses to the world are influenced by the exigencies of a particular situation. But most of the time we are like the investor or the architecture buff, with our central activities continuously conditioning our perceptions of persons, places, and events. Our way of life is not simply something we bring to situations; over time, our way of life develops its own power and momentum in defining situations and our responses to them.

So a heavy drinker arrives for an informal party at a friend's house. While the other guests scan the room to seek out the host or to notice the decor or the food, the heavy drinker immediately searches for the bar and winces if it is poorly equipped. And as guests begin to circulate to see who else has arrived, the heavy drinker notices one crony who has on occasion joined him for a few rounds at the neighborhood bar, and an eagle-eyed friend of his brother's, one who's sure to report disapprovingly on how much drinking went on at the party.

When we speak of the momentum of a way of life, we are using a convenient label to refer to the cumulative impact of many long-cultivated and interrelated habits of mind, heart, soul, and body. For most of us, it is only when we are contemplating a serious change in some central activity that we come to consciously realize the momentum the activity has acquired.

We feel that we ought to be able to accomplish this one limited change without our lives falling apart, but the change turns out to be not so limited after all. Changing our type of career or our style of social life, deciding to do some serious reading instead of watching TV, to worry less about ourselves and more about others, to eat less, to save more—all these require changes in all sorts of other routines, attitudes, and ways of behaving. Even if we desire the end result of the proposed change—higher salary, trimmer figure, more security, a better quality of life—the change suddenly seems far more disruptive than we could have imagined. At this point we may feel in the grip of some alien opposing power that is trying to prevent us from doing what we rationally want to do.

But the obstacle is not in truth an alien power. It is our deeply rooted habit-bound self opposing the fragile reed of a new desire to be other than who or what we have been. And the more genuine our desire to change, the more tense and intense the conflict. To others, our difficulty in making the decision to change may seem puzzling, for why would we not want to commit to a change that we say is attractive and that has obvious advantages over our present situation?

This perplexity brings us directly to the puzzling quality of the heavy drinker's behavior. It is not that some innerspring of self-control is broken, but that for the heavy drinker the decision to drink or not to drink is far more than a matter of reaching or not reaching for a bottle or a glass. Like any of us contemplating a major change in a central activity, the heavy drinker cannot simply reshape his or her life at will. Internal and external factors—bodily constitution and age, intellect and education, cultural and ethnic norms, economic and domestic circumstances—limit one's potential for change and one's alternatives.

Of course, neither are we helpless to reshape our lives in significant ways. What I have to do (if not I, *who?*) is to take responsibility within the limits imposed by my life for selecting and achieving realistic goals. There are no guarantees, no techniques or treatments that assuredly work for all. This is basic common sense, not anything peculiar to heavy drinkers.

In talking about heavy drinking in this way, I am simply translating into everyday language the key concepts of the recent research literature. Much of what I have been saying was summarized, for example, over ten years ago in the following terms:

> There is no single entity which can be defined as alcoholism.
>
> There is no clear dichotomy between either alcoholics and non-alcoholics, or between prealcoholics and nonprealcoholics even though individuals may have differing susceptibility to both the use of alcohol and the development of alcohol problems as a result of genetic, physiological, psychological, and sociocultural factors.
>
> The . . . sequence [in which] adverse consequences [develop] appears to be highly variable.
>
> There is no evidence to date for a basic biological process that predisposes an individual toward [abuse] of alcohol.
>
> The empirical evidence suggests that alcohol problems are reversible.
>
> Alcohol problems are typically interrelated with other life problems.[2]

Unfortunately for the sake of the general public, scientists and researchers often conduct their discussions in almost unreadable technical language. For example, in the journals published for specialists, one may read that:

> alcohol-related problems [are] understood best as behavioral disorders which are established and maintained as a result of the unique, direct, and reciprocal interactions of behavioral, discriminative, incentive, and social elements, all of which function with varying degrees of cognitive mediation. Within the framework of this multivariate approach, it is assumed that each of these elements or dimensions is interactive and yet each is sufficiently discrete to preserve its own, albeit cognitively mediated, locus of control. Such a multivariate approach permits an assessment

of both the nature and the extent of the involvement of each of
the elements (behavioral, discriminative, incentive, and social),
which are variously integrated within the overall cognitive func-
tioning of the individual and which account for that person's "al-
coholismic" behavior.[3]

This arcane language tells us essentially the same things that I
have been explaining in everyday language: there is no one
cause of alcoholism; alcohol abuse is the outcome of a range
of physical, personal, and social characteristics that together
predispose a person to drink to excess; and episodes of heavy
drinking are triggered by immediate events in a person's life.

From the basic perspective we have been outlining, specific
elements of a heavy drinker's way of life are not symptoms of
a disease but rather clues to the character of that life. For example, morning drinking has been labeled a symptom of alcoholism. Viewed against our cultural norm of not drinking
early in the day, morning drinking is indeed a noteworthy
event. And it is a behavior far more typical of heavy drinkers
than social drinkers.

But although morning drinking is a meaningful clue about
a drinker's way of life, to call it a symptom imputes a disease
and connotes a medical phenomenon. By way of analogy: If
we heard a person frequently discussing business over breakfast, we would not call this activity a "symptom" of an ambitious commitment to business. But we might consider this
breach of cultural norms regarding polite breakfast conversation to be a reliable sign of some significant dimensions of the
speaker's way of life.

A similar point needs to be made about secret drinking,
which has also been labeled a symptom of alcoholism. Again
the very word *symptom* takes a nonmedical event and turns it
into a medical one. Yet few of us broadcast our failings and
shortcomings; rather, we tend to be secretive about any of our
activities that we feel deviate from social norms, especially if—
despite our behavior—we still believe in those norms. It seems

perfectly natural and human that some combination of shame, guilt, or prudence leads us to hide our nonconforming behavior. The tendency of heavy drinkers to hide their drinking is thus a fully intelligible expression of human propensities.

And what we hide from others we also sometimes try to hide from ourselves. Self-deception is a universally welcome solace that everyone engages in at times to maintain self-respect.[4] Denial may not be an ideal way to handle life's problems, but neither is it a symptom of a disease. Yes, drinkers often deny their problems, but as one committee of researchers put it: "Of course, the problem of facing worrying facts is not unique to drinking. If someone is frightened or ashamed of his behavior, he is likely to hide or deny what he is doing; this is an understandable defensive strategy."[5]

The drinker's motives, then, are no different than anyone else's, though they often lead to self-destructive ends. Like all of us, drinkers struggle to defend and rationalize their choices in life. The scenarios, motives, and defense mechanisms are infinitely many and various.

Consider, for example, a husband who is hurt and angered by what he perceives as his wife's indifference toward him. In this situation one man might become visibly angry and confront his wife with his grievances. But another man might feel himself unable to speak out; fear, guilt, low self-esteem or other emotions may block an overt confrontation. Instead, he may adopt evasive, ultimately unconstructive ways of handling the situation. He may simply sulk, and let his moroseness be his sullen revenge. Or he may seek the company of other women. Or he may get drunk and then act out his anger, hiding behind the culturally sanctioned excuse that people are not fully responsible for their behavior when they are drunk. This evasion of responsibility helps appease his conscience; he is contrite when sober and claims he "hardly knows what he is doing" when drunk. He even claims a certain sympathy for his propensity—eventually his "disease" or his "compulsion"—to drink and to lose control of himself. Thus he comes to see himself as the victim, even though it is his wife who has to endure his drunken outbursts.

Some people catch themselves in the act of dodging their problems and difficulties and call a halt to their evasive tactics. But at times any of us may find it easier to avoid a problem than to face it squarely. We find ourselves repeating the avoidance activities to maintain the evasion, and slowly the avoidance activities take on a momentum of their own. Eventually, the avoidance pattern becomes easier and easier, more and more spontaneously favored in response to a wide variety of threatening or anxiety-producing situations. Over time, an avoidance response like overeating or gambling or drinking may in itself become a focal activity for a small number of people.

Thus there is no one story of how people become heavy drinkers. Nor is there some mysterious demon afoot—at each point the heavy drinker's conduct is an intelligible version of normal cognitive and emotional behaviors.

## Willpower and Responsibility

Once we view heavy drinking as a central activity, we can better appreciate how deeply interwoven drinking is in the fabric of the drinker's life. We will no longer try to detach the drinking from the drinker's entire way of being in the world:

> Anyone who has had experience with the treatment of alcoholism will realize that the drinking problem does not exist in isolation. . . . [I]t is a *person* who is coming for help, with an essential sense of being a person with various troubles and perplexities which exist in their own right, and which may predate the excessive drinking, or cause it, or intertwine with it, or exacerbate it.[6]

To focus only on the drinking behavior, in isolation from all else, is to miss the point that a central activity reverberates throughout a person's way of life.

Thus for a heavy drinker to make a major change in his drinking patterns requires a reconstruction of his way of life. The drinker must learn over time to see the world in different terms, to cultivate new values and interests, to find or create new physical and social settings, to develop new relationships, to devise new ways of behaving in those new relationships and settings.[7] Many heavy drinkers do this on their own initiative, "maturing out" of heavy drinking with no professional help. They are often aided by the moral support of others around them. Often the process is closely linked to a change, perhaps fortuitous, in a drinker's life circumstances, such as a new job, a change in domestic or personal relationships, or the greater self-discipline that often emerges as one grows older. Also important are changes in others' attitudes and responses to the drinker. A person's way of life, after all, is not an isolated, purely individual affair but is to a great extent responsive to the behaviors of others.

The drinker's development of new attitudes, new values, and new skills cannot be a matter of making an isolated decision or of mere willpower. But resoluteness and willpower are a necessary first step. That willpower alone may not be sufficient to achieve the desired goal should not mislead anyone into discounting willpower or into assuming that the willpower of heavy drinkers has been irreparably impaired by alcohol.

On this particular issue Vaillant, for example, overreacts and oversimplifies when he says that "willpower is inferior to behavior modification," that is, that the drinker's will to change must be continually reinforced by a program of incentives and disincentives intended to reliably condition the drinker's choices.[8] Vaillant is correct insofar as merely to announce firmly to oneself and others that one is resolved to change is not enough. But inner resolve is not inferior as a force for reconstruction; choice is not magically effective, but neither is it a mere illusion.[9] One can insist that a drinker can and must assume some responsibility for change, even while admitting that this commitment alone will not turn the tide.

Thus we must put aside both the old simplistic moralism, which taught that a sincere resolve was enough, and the loss-of-control hypothesis, which viewed each failure of willpower as proof that the drinker's will had been incapacitated by disease. Let us instead view willpower as we do the signing of a contract. Signing a contract does not get the job done, but neither do we think that contracts are pointless, meaningless statements. They are necessary and important elements within a sequence of events that may or may not result in the fulfillment of the intended transaction.

In sum, any efforts that heavy drinkers take to change their drinking activities must be predicated on an acceptance of personal responsibility. This resolve, in turn, must be followed by actions intended to achieve a reshaping of their way of life that fosters change and precludes situations that frustrate the will to change. And because heavy drinking as a central activity has many meanings for the drinker, the reconstruction of life must go well beyond eliminating the drinking activity to building new and satisfying ways of meeting life's challenges.

## Conclusions

If we genuinely understand the meaning of heavy drinking as a central activity, we will feel compassion for chronic drinkers, their struggles to cope with human stresses and strains. There is no reason to see heavy drinking as a symptom of illness, a sign of persistent evil, or the mark of conscienceless will. Rarely do people wickedly choose a destructive or self-destructive way of life. On the contrary, we shape our lives day by day, crisis by crisis, often only in retrospect able to see the pattern that was evolving. We each share the propensity to choose opportunistically when under stress. So, on a series of occasions, a drinker chooses what seems the lesser evil, the temporarily easier compromise, without a clear appreciation of the long-run implications.

If our righteous condemnation is not in order, neither is our cooperation in excusing heavy drinkers or helping them evade responsibility for change. Compassion, constructive aid, and the respect manifest in expecting a person to act responsibly—these are usually the reasonable basic attitudes to take when confronting a particular heavy drinker who is in trouble. The drinker is responsible for paying attention, for caring, for taking individual measures, often small ones that, like the small rudder on a large ship, are intended to crucially redirect a life. There is no more validity to putting the entire burden of successful change on the drinker's goodwill than in absolving him of all responsibility as though he were helpless.

Clearly, more than compassion is in order. Heavy drinkers need moral and psychological support, sound advice about their situation, and help in self-understanding. In the next chapter we will apply our new perspective directly to the issue of helping individual heavy drinkers. And in the last chapter I will discuss several social policies that could prevent or curtail heavy drinking.

One may feel a certain frustration that no one has found one single explanation of one uniform ailment. On the other hand, perhaps the single most positive outcome of the new perspective on alcohol abuse is that we no longer restrict our efforts to achieving an all-or-none outcome with a relatively small proportion of heavy drinkers, the supposed "true alcoholics." We can devise ways of helping a far wider needful population and we can do so with greater realism and flexibility. We can also address the social aspects of drinking, and the class, ethnic, cultural, economic, and religious dimensions. The very complexity of the causes and courses of alcohol abuse encourages us to draw upon the insights and methods of many disciplines. This redefinition of the problem and our approach to it thus offers hope, though it does not promise easy answers.

## Notes

1. Holden, "Is Alcoholism Treatment Effective?" (1987b), 23. See also Caddy, "A Multivariate Approach to Restricted Drinking" (1982).
2. These six points excerpted from Pattison, Sobell, and Sobell, *Emerging Concepts of Alcohol Dependence* (1977), 189–90. See also Room, "Sociological Aspects of the Disease Concept of Alcoholism" (1983); P. Davies, "Does Treatment Work?" (1985).
3. Caddy (1982), 276.
4. Fingarette, "Alcoholism and Self-Deception" (1985b).
5. *Alcohol and Alcoholism* (1979), 119.
6. *Alcohol and Alcoholism* (1979), 120.
7. A key finding of a survey of treatment professionals is that 80 percent mentioned "social and personal adjustment" and changes in family, social, and work-related situations as criteria of success in dealing with alcohol problems; see P. Davies (1985), 162–63.
8. Vaillant, *The Natural History of Alcoholism* (1983), 191. For a typical account that describes but underplays the need for the alcoholic to recognize his problems and take responsibility for his drinking, see Schuckit, "Treatment of Alcoholism in Office and Outpatient Settings" (1985b), 309–10.
9. For example, although writing from different theoretical perspectives, each of the following influential authorities affirms the importance of the drinker's assuming responsibility and making a personal commitment to change: Schuckit (1985b), 309; Marlatt, "Psychosocial Perspectives on Alcoholism Treatment and the Process of Recovery" (1982); *Alcohol and Alcoholism* (1979), 56; Orford, "Alcoholism" (1976).

# CHAPTER 6

# Helping the Heavy Drinker

As we saw in Chapter 4, traditional alcoholism treatment programs tend to view individual differences among heavy drinkers as largely irrelevant to the treatment regimen, though these differences are acknowledged to affect rates of recovery. In theory at least, the disease-oriented programs affirm that all their patients are suffering from the same disease, an ailment so powerful that it overwhelms individual differences.

In contrast, the central premise of all the approaches described in this chapter is that heavy drinkers are a widely diverse group and that an appreciation of individual differences is fundamental to any efforts designed to help alcohol abusers. Therefore, no one method of treatment or help can be expected to prove effective for all drinkers. People who seek help need a program tailored to their personal characteristics (age, sex, marital status, socioeconomic and occupational class, cultural background), their particular drinking patterns and behavior, and their motives for drinking or ceasing to drink.

Thus before initiating any type of counseling or therapy,

one would want to understand the drinker's personal history and situation. Among the relevant questions: On what occasions, in what settings, and with what frequency does this person drink heavily? In what kind of moods, and with what sorts of expectations? How long has this person been drinking heavily? With what physical and psychological effects? What purposes does drinking serve for this person?

Furthermore, because drinking is a central activity interwoven throughout the fabric of the drinker's life, these new approaches do not view the excision or suppression of drinking activity as a realistic or sufficient goal. The aim is to help the drinker begin to develop an integrated and satisfying way of life in which heavy drinking will no longer be central.

Most of the techniques described in this chapter are still being field-tested. Carefully done studies and experiments have been sufficiently confirmatory to justify optimism, but not all the needed data are in, and several studies have raised important questions and controversies. Thus while I am cautiously sympathetic to these newer approaches, their efficacy has not yet been fully demonstrated. I believe that the evidence entitles us to hope, but at this stage we cannot leap from hope to certainty.

## Matching

One general strategy that opens up many opportunities for individualized help is *matching*, the principle of pairing drinkers with the kind of program best suited to their personal history and way of life.[1] Matching seems a rather commonsense idea, but it also may resolve the troublesome issue raised in Chapter 4: that the results of many programs do not exceed the rate of natural improvement because their success with some kinds of drinkers and their relative ineffectiveness with other kinds causes a "statistical washout." As we have seen, "if the *same* treatment is indiscriminately applied to all patients, the results on balance do not improve upon the results achieved [merely by giving] advice."[2] The matching principle suggests that the overall success rates might improve if drinkers seeking help were carefully paired with the most suitable program.

The ultimate applications of matching would entail the creation of a vast database derived from many large-scale studies that measured the effectiveness of different treatment regimens with specific categories of heavy drinkers. For example, for each drinker in these studies, the following kinds of information would be collected:

personal characteristics (age, sex, occupation, and socioeconomic status)

drinking history and patterns (length, frequency, motives)

assessment of physical and mental health on admission to treatment

nature of the treatment (inpatient or outpatient, length of the program, techniques used, style and personality of therapist, degree of structure)

drinking behavior at followup (abstinence, moderate drinking, or heavy drinking; amount and frequency of drinking)

overall health and behavior at followup (job stability, days of work missed, police or domestic incidents).

All this information would be statistically analyzed to produce a menu of probabilities indicating which treatment programs best achieve which outcomes with which kinds of drinkers.

The creation of such an immense and detailed database is still years away. And while the concept is gaining adherents in the research community, one careful review of the literature on matching concludes that the results—in both alcoholism treatment and psychotherapy in general—seem little better than those that common sense would have afforded.[3] Some of the objections and criticisms, however, may be resolved as clinical and statistical techniques reach a higher level of refinement.

The potential of matching is hinted at by a study that correlated drinkers' performance at followup with two measures of the style of the treatment they had received.[4] The treatment program under study had not intentionally tried to match client and therapist—that is, the matches or mismatches detected by the research study had occurred naturally during the program, which involved counseling, psychotherapy, and psychodrama.

Ninety-four diagnosed alcoholics who had completed the program were extensively interviewed and tested twelve to sixteen months later. At this followup, the drinkers' drinking behavior was rated on a 4-point scale: no improvement, some improvement, mostly abstinent, fully abstinent. Drinkers in the latter two categories were considered to be recovered.

At the followup each drinker was also rated on a 4-point scale, Conceptual Level, devised by the researcher as a general indicator of personality:

1. poorly socialized, egocentric, impulsive, cognitively simple
2. dependent and compliant
3. independent, questioning, self-assertive
4. interdependent, empathic, and cognitively complex.

All the program's therapists were also assigned a rating on this scale. (As one might expect, none of the therapists were rated at the lowest level; but a match between drinker and therapist at level 1 would not have been desirable.)

Finally, each drinker's aftercare setting was rated as high or low in structure, depending on the amount of contact and counseling the drinker had had since completing treatment.

These data were than analyzed to determine how strongly

recovery was correlated with matches or mismatches between the drinker's Conceptual Level and the therapist's Conceptual Level, and with matches or mismatches between the drinker's Conceptual Level and the structuredness of the aftercare setting. The variances were large enough to be statistically significant:

|  | Recovery Rate |
|---|---|
| Drinker and therapist matched | 70% |
| Drinker and therapist mismatched | 50% |
| Drinker and setting matched | 71% |
| Drinker and setting mismatched | 49% |
| Drinker, therapist, and setting matched | 77% |
| Drinker, therapist, and setting mismatched | 38% |

The comparative advantage in recovery rates for the "match" groups is quite impressive, although clearly these few simple measures of compatibility merely skim the surface. But results such as these tend to confirm commonsense propositions about the relationship between people's motivational style and their need for more or less structure, or about the advantages and disadvantages of personal compatibility between therapist and client.

## Individualized Behavioral Approaches

Many of the new approaches are called behavioral because they consider heavy drinking as an activity—rather than an ailment—that plays a part in a way of life.[5] The word *behavioral*, however, should not mislead anyone into thinking of the crude, now obsolete methods that relied on behavioral conditioning after the pattern of Pavlov. While dogs may be trained to salivate on cue, human beings are far more complex, and "there is not and never has been any convincing evidence for the unconscious, automatic mechanism in the conditioning of adult human beings."[6]

Further, these new behavioral approaches should not be confused with other older forms of classical behavioral methodology. For example, at one time the administration of an electric shock immediately after a drinker took a drink was considered a theoretically promising application of operant conditioning. In the absence of evidence supporting its long-term effectiveness, this method has been abandoned, though chemical aversion programs (Schick-Shadel, for example) that rely on the same negative-reinforcement principle are still widespread.[7]

The new behavioral methods under consideration here, in addition to matching, appear under a variety of names and labels: Individualized Behavior Therapy, broad-spectrum therapy, Relapse Prevention Therapy, behavioral self-control strategies, and so on. Too, so many variants are emerging that we can give only an impressionistic sketch here.[8]

Individualized Behavior Therapy, for example, emphasizes the analysis of the individual heavy drinker's way of life and the role drinking plays in it. Drinker and therapist identify the settings and circumstances in which drinking goes on and then jointly try to devise new practical ways of responding to those situations, new ways of living that avoid such situations, and new ways of addressing the social, situational, and physical motivations to drink. One technique is for the drinker and therapist to set up a realistic drinking setting—perhaps a room fixed up like a public bar—that allows the drinker to practice new ways of handling invitations and opportunities to drink.[9] Or the drinker is asked to imagine a situation in which he or she would typically drink, but to role-play the situation of saying no. The roles and the solutions are worked out by the drinker and the therapist to fit the drinker's particular situation, capacities, and opportunities.

Other so-called broad-spectrum approaches combine advice, counseling, teaching, role-playing, aversive therapy, and self-analysis. In one successful therapy for a young man who fit the medical criteria for alcohol dependence (alcoholism) the selected techniques included: teaching him better ways to conduct an argument with his wife, encouraging him to pay off his debts, counseling him to learn a marketable skill after going back to school, and carefully instructing him about how to make decisions about drinking in a variety of contexts.[10]

Another important approach to helping heavy drinkers is called Relapse Prevention. The key idea is the recognition that a commitment to changing the way one lives is a learning process, a process in which slips and errors may occur in the early phases but should become less frequent as learning progresses. Thus, instead of the do-or-die attitude of the disease-oriented programs, with their stress on total and permanent abstention as the only alternative to disaster, Relapse Prevention gives drinkers specific practical help in avoiding slips, but also in overcoming slips and learning from mistakes. This approach is supported by experimental and theoretical research into the dynamics of self-change viewed as a gradual learning process rather than instant and total conversion.[11]

It is too soon to tell how confidently these various techniques can be applied. For the attempt to help a person reshape a way of life is a chancy affair. The old way of life has, by its very nature, a powerful momentum that staunchly resists change. Moreover, whether the drinker's family, friends, and co-workers are aware of it or not, they may be acting in ways that thwart the drinker's efforts to change. Even though the intimates of the drinker may not do the drinking, they are integral parts of the way of life that centers around drinking. In some cases family members and friends are unconsciously a part of the problem and not merely victims of it. Today some disease-oriented programs also involve the drinker's family in efforts to understand and improve family dynamics, although this is somewhat inconsistent with the premise that alcoholism is a disease afflicting the drinker.

## Flexible Measures of Success

One of the major, and most controversial, implications of these new approaches is that it is totally unrealistic to view a drinker's efforts to change his or her way of life as an all-or-none affair. Instead of looking only at changes in drinking behavior, one needs to look at all the changes that the drinker is trying to make. And instead of judging success in changing drinking behavior solely on the criterion of total abstinence, one looks to see if there is a substantial reduction in the number of drinking days a month, or a major reduction in the amount typically drunk at any one time, or a marked reduction in days off the job, or of weeks in the hospital, or of fights or squabbles with others. Any of these outcomes can constitute a significant and highly desirable change, even if the drinker still drinks or even drinks heavily.

The measurement of such outcomes and the acknowledgment of the achievements they represent do not mean that these outcomes need be set as goals. It is not inconsistent or unconstructive to set abstinence as a goal, but to measure intermediate events that show a reduction in drinking or a decrease in problems caused by drinking. Conversely, once a drinker's overall quality of life is used as one of several measures of success, total abstinence in and of itself is not necessarily a sign of success.

In many cases a heavy drinker's quality of life is improved by abstention, but there is mixed evidence about the effects of abstinence on this score. Merely ceasing to drink may cause serious psychological or stress-related physical problems if other aspects of the drinker's way of life have not also changed.[12] One cannot simply and without consequences forsake a central activity, abandon a preferred coping strategy, or disable a defense mechanism—however costly it has proven to be.

Thus to note only whether a heavy drinker achieves abstinence or not is to miss a large part of the picture. If after treatment the drinker takes an occasional drink or develops a pattern of abstinence over most of the year with perhaps two or three scattered episodes of heavy drinking, these significant changes should not be deemed failures.

New definitions of success also affect the evaluation of disease-oriented treatments. A recent large-scale study of Antabuse, for example, showed Antabuse to produce no significant increase in the rate of continuous complete abstinence over twelve months.[13] Assessed by the criterion of total abstinence, then, this study was merely the latest in a series that have shown Antabuse to be a failure. But these researchers also measured the number of days during the year on which the nonabstinent drinkers drank, and they found that those drinkers who had been prescribed the regular Antabuse regimen drank on significantly fewer days than the others. The interpretation of this result is difficult because other factors were also associated with reduced drinking. But, surely, if heavy drinkers will continue to drink, it is preferable that they do so on significantly fewer occasions.

Similarly, a four-year followup study of some 780 alcoholics in eight alcoholism treatment centers reported that while about 30 percent of the subjects achieved long-term abstinence, significant decreases were found in the rate of drinking (down by 70 percent), physical dependence symptoms (down by 60 percent), and problem drinking (down from over 90 percent to 54 percent).[14] To ignore such outcomes or to place the less frequent, lighter drinkers and the more frequent, heavier drinkers in the single category of "failure to abstain" is counterproductive, both for the drinkers who are trying to improve their lives and for researchers who are seeking better ways of helping heavy drinkers.

Another part of the process of redefining measures of success is redefining measures of problem drinking. If a former heavy drinker still drinks, but much less than before, and also gets a divorce, should the divorce be tabulated as an alcohol-related domestic problem? Perhaps the divorce was part of the drinker's solution to deeper underlying problems. Thus the notion that certain events (divorce, quitting a job, leaving town) are per se evidence of problems oversimplifies the meaning of the event in the life of a particular individual.

Inevitably, the new flexibility opens up much room for disagreement. Once one discards the dichotomy of abstinent-nonabstinent, one faces difficult distinctions in deciding which behaviors, attitudes, and events are to be considered positive outcomes for a particular drinker. For example, one research team, in analyzing the results of treatment of a large number of heavy drinkers, used the category "returning to normal drinking."[15] The team was criticized in several quarters because the criteria for this category were implausibly high: individuals were classified as "returning to normal" even if they were having as many as six or seven drinks a day and had in the preceding month as many as two blackouts, two days missed from work because of alcohol, and four episodes of morning drinking. For Vaillant, among others, "even one of these symptoms in a *year* would be considered evidence of alcohol abuse."[16]

A reanalysis of the data segregated all those originally classified as "returning to normal drinking" into two groups: those showing any physical symptoms or alcohol-related adverse consequences at the followups and those showing no symptoms or adverse consequences related to drinking. Slightly more than half of those originally classified as normal drinkers under the original, more generous definition showed no physical symptoms or alcohol-related problems either at the

eighteen-month or four-year followups, despite their continuing to drink. After four years, 12 percent of those who were
physically dependent at admission to treatment were nonabstinent and yet drank without any problems, as did 30 percent of those who at admission were somewhat physically dependent.[17] Such figures, which are broadly consistent with
the ranges reported in other studies, suggest that—contrary
to the orthodox position of A.A. and other disease-oriented
approaches—physical dependency does not rule out a return
to moderate drinking.

The discovery that at least some heavy drinkers are able to
drink in moderation has also sparked a bitter controversy
about whether, at least for some drinkers, a form of moderated or controlled drinking might be preferable to abstinence
as a goal.

## Controlled Drinking

*Controlled drinking* has become the umbrella term for the
notion that abstinence need not be the only reasonable goal
for the heavy drinker seeking help.[18] One study, for example,
compared a treatment program that was abstinence-oriented
with another that had controlled drinking as its goal.[19] Judged
by the criterion of total abstinence, the two approaches were
equally successful: about one third of each group remained
abstinent for a year after treatment. But among those subjects
who did not maintain abstinence, the differences were strik-
ing. On an overall index of posttreatment drinking, which
used pretreatment behavior as a baseline, the drinkers in each
group were roughly comparable directly after treatment, at
about the 50 percent level. By the third month after the program, the average level of drinking for those in the abstinence-
oriented group had climbed to 70 percent of their pretreatment drinking level, while the group that had been taught

strategies for controlled drinking were at about the 20 percent level. By six months, the respective figures were about 50 percent and 5 percent, and at twelve months about 35 percent and 10 percent. Thus, over time the controlled-drinking group on average reduced their drinking far more than the abstinence group.

The fear prevalent among alcoholism treatment professionals and staff is that controlled drinking may all too easily give way to uncontrolled drinking. Some have called the adoption of controlled drinking as a treatment goal "dangerous and irresponsible." [20] The most virulent opponents have publicly stated that even the publication of scientific studies on the possibility of controlled drinking can "literally kill alcoholics." [21]

The controversy began in 1962, when D. L. Davies called attention to the accumulation of reports on diagnosed alcoholics who had shifted to controlled drinking. [22] Davies was sharply criticized; an unprecedented seventeen commentaries were published by the journal that had originally printed his article, and critical remarks were widely published in the press. An even more excoriating response, including a hostile and dramatic press conference called by the National Council on Alcoholism, was prompted in 1976 when an extensive national study reviewed the rapidly growing literature on controlled drinking and added confirmatory results. [23] Unfortunately, legitimate criticism of the study was lost in the barrage of condemnation, with some declaring the report dangerous or undeserving of notice and others wondering aloud if the report should have been suppressed.

In between these two battles in the war over controlled drinking, in 1972, Mark Sobell and Linda Sobell issued their groundbreaking report detailing the successful results of their elaborate and carefully evaluated program of controlled drinking. [24] A decade's worth of reasonable debate about the Sobells' work exploded into controversy in 1982 when Mary

Pendery and her coauthors published a highly critical review, which appeared in *Science* and was widely reported in the press.[25] The fireworks led to the appointment of a scientific commission to review the Sobells' study and, because the Sobells had received federal funds, a congressional staff investigation. The final reports of both the commission and the investigation defended the integrity of the Sobells' work.

Pendery's study itself was subsequently criticized at length by other researchers for having cited data out of context.[26] For example, Pendery stressed the grim fact that four of the subjects the Sobells had reported as successful controlled drinkers had died within ten years after completing the program; the resumption of heavy drinking was suspected as a contributing cause in these deaths. But Pendery failed to mention that in the equivalent comparison group, which received orthodox abstinence-oriented treatment, six subjects had died within the ten-year period. Placed in context, then, the mortality rate for the controlled drinkers showed that controlled drinking has its risks and failures, but that it may prove to be a significantly more successful method than abstinence for at least some drinkers.

One of the studies often cited to discount the usefulness of controlled drinking as a goal is a report on a controlled drinking program in which none of the subjects were successful.[27] But these subjects started with a poor prognosis, and the researchers took the worst day during a four-year followup period as the measure of success. Thus if a subject drank heavily once during the four years, he or she was counted as a total failure.

Despite the objections and criticisms, the literature on the numbers of former heavy drinkers who maintain moderate drinking continues to grow. A recent rigorous study reports that among socially adjusted former heavy drinkers, the majority were social drinkers rather than abstainers.[28] From the statistical data, researchers are beginning to extrapolate portraits of those drinkers who profit most from therapies that teach controlled drinking. For example, most heavy drinkers aged forty or older who show signs of severe physical dependence and who acknowledge themselves to be alcoholics tend to do better in programs aimed at abstinence, while heavy drinkers under forty who have moderate physical symptoms may be more successful if they learn to drink moderately rather than aim at abstention.[29]

These generalizations, of course, are quite broad, and a host of other factors must be taken into account in setting goals for an individual drinker. Indeed, within every statistical category (for instance, age, socioeconomic status, drinking history) a significant proportion of drinkers diverge from the overall pattern. Thus again, as we have noted before, no one approach can be expected to be effective for all heavy drinkers.

As we move from large-scale statistics to the individual drinker in search of help, four additional issues arise. First, putting aside the question of long-term effectiveness, some researchers who are sympathetic to controlled drinking stress the value of the concept in encouraging heavy drinkers to seek help and to moderate their drinking. In contrast, drinkers who have been misinformed that a return to moderation is always impossible, that the only alternative is total abstention, may be so discouraged or frightened by the immensity of the goal that they reject any thought of seeking help.[30]

Second, for heavy drinkers who are trying to address their problems, the concept of controlled drinking can have the salutary effect of acknowledging human fallibility. If backsliding is viewed as a normal event in the difficult effort to develop new habits, attitudes, and responses, then mistakes along the way are not viewed as devastating failures but as natural missteps in discovering a new path.

Third, at this time global conclusions about the practicability of controlled drinking as a goal are premature. We need to develop more specific and nuanced ways of categorizing, measuring, and discriminating different patterns of drinking and associated phenomena. It is simply too soon for us to know how to respond to qualified objections like the following: "We do not challenge the reports of Sobell and Sobell that individuals with alcohol dependence can become controlled drinkers, although even here the concept of controlled drinking needs elaboration. We do doubt, based on our own clinical experience and a review of the literature . . . that many gamma alcoholics with *significant* physical dependence can become controlled drinkers." [31]

Fourth, the question of what constitutes *controlled* drinking for a given drinker remains a point of controversy. Some researchers find *controlled* a misnomer for drinking that is still relatively heavy and erratic in frequency and duration.

Finally, it is worth noting that controlled drinking programs for problem drinkers are routinely available in other countries, especially the United Kingdom, Canada, and Norway. In the United Kingdom, for example, three-fourths of the clinics offer controlled drinking as an alternative. [32] But in our country, the ideological preoccupation with the disease concept of alcoholism has forestalled the establishment of programs with goals other than total abstinence. [33]

## Conclusions

The new perspective on heavy drinking suggests that all aspects of treatment—methods, goals, measures of success— must be carefully chosen to reflect the individual drinker and his or her way of life. For to alter one's drinking behavior is a complex achievement that often requires a difficult struggle to reorganize one's life and learn to live differently. But, as the data show, heavy drinkers who are motivated to change and who are persistent in the face of setbacks can change if they are given the appropriate tools and strategies for reshaping their lives.[34]

All the newer approaches also emphasize that the drinker must accept responsibility and play an active role in bringing about the desired change. No longer is the heavy drinker viewed as a victim of disease, a passive patient who will be treated by an expert: "In contrast with the disease model and its emphasis on the uncontrollable . . . self-control theorists have emphasized that the individual is capable of exercising control and assuming responsibility."[35] However, it seems equally crucial that heavy drinkers assume such responsibilities "without berating themselves for their role in creating these problems."[36] As one author puts it, heavy drinkers must learn to accept "[that] imperfection exists, that negative feelings will return, that slips will occur, and that insoluble problems and a sense of inadequate rewards will never disappear entirely. . . . [O]nly those who are willing to tolerate the uncertainty of a life without the addiction and who believe they can tolerate it will succeed in doing so."[37]

## Notes

1. On the general principle of matching, see Glaser, "Anybody Got a Match?" (1980); Glaser and Skinner, "Matching in the Real World" (1981).
2. Glaser (1980), 187.
3. Sells, "Matching Clients to Treatments" (1981).
4. McLachlan, "Therapy Strategies, Personality Orientation, and Recovery from Alcoholism" (1974).
5. On behavioral approaches in general, see Nathan, Marlatt, and Loberg, *Alcoholism* (1978); Hodgson, "Behaviour Therapy" (1976); Miller, *Behavioral Treatment of Alcoholism* (1976).
6. Brewer, "There Is No Convincing Evidence for Operant or Classical Conditioning in Adult Humans" (1974), 27. For a more

qualified review, see Siegel, "Classical Conditioning, Drug Tolerance and Drug Dependence" (1983).

7. On programs using negative reinforcement, see Nathan and Niaura, "Behavioral Assessment and Treatment of Alcoholism" (1985), 418–20 and 422; Marlatt, "The Controlled Drinking Controversy" (1983), 1102; Neuberger et al., "Replicable Abstinence Rates in an Alcoholism Treatment Program" (1982); Lemere and Voegtlin, "An Evaluation of the Aversion Treatment of Alcoholism" (1950).

8. For descriptions of various individualized behavioral therapies, see Nathan and Niaura (1985), 430–42; M. Sobell and L. Sobell, *Individualized Behavioral Therapy for Alcoholics* (1972); Marlatt, "Relapse Prevention" (1985); Glaser (1980); Glaser and Skinner (1981). On related approaches that focus on environmental factors, see Peele, *The Meaning of Addiction* (1985); Ogborne, Sobell, and Sobell, "The Significance of Environmental Factors for the Design and the Evaluation of Alcohol Treatment Programs" (1985).

9. M. Sobell and L. Sobell (1972), 72.

10. L. Sobell, "Behavioral Treatment of Outpatient Problem Drinkers [case no. 1]" (1982).

11. For a full account of the theory and methods, see Marlatt and Gordon, *Relapse Prevention* (1985).

12. See Heather and Robertson, *Controlled Drinking* (1981), 133–38.

13. Fuller et al., "Disulfiram Treatment of Alcoholism" (1986).

14. Polich, Armor, and Braiker, *The Course of Alcoholism* (1980), 64 and 171.

15. On the criteria used by Armor, Polich, and Stambul, *Alcoholism and Treatment* (1976), see Polich, Armor, and Braiker (1980), 63 (table 3.29).

16. Vaillant, *The Natural History of Alcoholism* (1983), 233.

17. Polich, Armor, and Braiker (1980), 63 and 60–61.

18. For a recent review of the debates, see Roizen, "The Great Controlled-Drinking Controversy" (1987). For a full-scale review sympathetic to controlled drinking, see Heather and Robertson (1981); Gottheil et al., "Alcoholics' Patterns of Controlled Drinking" (1973).

19. Marlatt (1983), 1103–4.

20. Orford and Edwards, *Alcoholism—A Comparison of Treatment and Advice* (1977), 117.

21. Royce, *Alcohol Problems and Alcoholism* (1981); see also Hingson, Scotch, and Goldman, "Impact of the 'Rand Report' on Alcoholics, Treatment Personnel and Boston Residents" (1977), 2066.

22. D. Davies, "Normal Drinking in Recovered Alcohol Addicts" (1962).

23. The report was Armor, Polich, and Stambul (1976), and the response to it is described in Heather and Robertson (1981), 58.

24. M. Sobell and L. Sobell (1972).

25. Pendery, Maltzman, and West, "Controlled Drinking by Alcoholics?" (1982). For a sample of the press coverage, see Boffey, "Alcoholism Study Under New Attack" (1982).

26. Peele, unpublished letter (1986); Marlatt (1983); M. Sobell and L. Sobell, "The Aftermath of Heresy" (1984).

27. Ewing and Rouse, "Failure of an Experimental Treatment Programme to Inculcate Controlled Drinking in Alcoholics" (1976).

28. Nordstrom and Berglund, "A Prospective Study of Successful Long-Term Adjustment in Alcohol Dependence" (1987). Similarly, Orford and Edwards (1977), 105, note that "controlled drinking amongst former alcoholics or excessive drinkers is far from being an uncommon phenomenon, but is rather one of the major alternative treatment outcomes." Pattison, "The Selection of Treatment Modalities for the Alcoholic Patient" (1985), 262–70, reviews the evidence that many different kinds of moderate drinking patterns are consistent with important betterment of the quality of life. See also Pattison, Sobell, and Sobell, *Emerging Concepts of Alcohol Dependence* (1977), 120–41; Orford, Oppenheimer, and Edwards, "Abstinence or Control" (1976); Pomerleau, Pertschuk, and Stinnent, "A Critical Examination of Some Current Assumptions in the Treatment of Alcoholism" (1976); Popham and Schmidt, "Some Factors Affecting the Likelihood of Moderate Drinking by Treated Alcoholics" (1976).

29. See Armor, "The RAND Reports and the Analysis of Relapse" (1980); Orford, "A Comparison of Alcoholics Whose Drinking Is Totally Uncontrolled and Those Whose Drinking Is Mainly Controlled" (1973); Polich, Armor, and Braiker (1980), 184; Nordstrom and Berglund (1987), 101.

30. On the ways in which abstinence discourages heavy drinkers

from seeking help, see M. Sobell and L. Sobell (1972); Reinert, "The Concept of Alcoholism as a Disease" (1968); Pattison, "A Critique of Alcoholism Treatment Concepts with Special Reference to Abstinence" (1966); Brunner-Orne, "Comment on 'Normal' Drinking in Recovered Alcohol Addicts" (1963); Gerard, Sanger, and Wile, "The Abstinent Alcoholic" (1962). On the many important possibilities of improvement that the goal of abstinence denies drinkers, see Pattison (1985), 262–70.

31. Kissin, "The Disease Concept of Alcoholism" (1983), 107.

32. Rush and Ogborne, "Acceptability of Nonabstinence Treatment Goals Among Alcoholism Treatment Programs" (1986).

33. Peele, "The Cultural Context of Psychological Approaches to Alcoholism" (1984), 1342; Peele (1985), 37–45; Marlatt (1983), 1101.

34. L. Sobell and M. Sobell, "Alcohol Treatment Outcome Evaluation Methodology" (1982), 315.

35. Marlatt, "Psychosocial Perspectives on Alcoholism Treatment and the Process of Recovery" (1982), 8. See also Edwards et al., *Alcohol and Alcoholism* (1979), 56.

36. Brickman et al., "Models of Helping and Coping" (1982), 372.

37. Peele (1985), 156.

CHAPTER 7

# Social Policies to Prevent
# and Control Heavy Drinking

In addressing the prevalence of alcohol abuse in our country, programs that offer assistance and guidance to individual drinkers are obviously only part of the solution. Clearly, society will never be able to persuade all the drinkers who need help to seek it out. And if even a fourth of those who need help were to seek it, the therapeutic resources—staff, administration, and public health or private insurance funding—would be strained well past their limits. Furthermore, as we noted earlier, most of the drinkers who encounter serious problems associated with alcohol are not long-term heavy drinkers. Programs have generally not been designed to assist these problem drinkers; nor can we expect these drinkers to seek help in time, before they fall into trouble.

Thus, in addition to encouraging heavy drinkers to seek help and providing the most effective kinds of services, we need to consider how best to prevent people from becoming heavy drinkers in the first place and how to discourage ex-

133

cessive consumption by people who have already started abusing alcohol. Since we now know that even the heaviest of drinkers do moderate their drinking in response to such disincentives as increases in cost or inconvenience (see Chapter 2), we can begin to contemplate new social policies specifically intended to depress consumption.

The new perspective on heavy drinking as a way of life, and not a faceless disease, opens up new avenues for educational, legal, economic, and political measures that could influence the choices of current and prospective heavy drinkers by affecting their perceptions of the short-term and long-term costs and benefits of drinking.

At the same time, we must be realistic. No set of social policies, however broad or imaginative, will eliminate alcohol abuse because "drinking is an important and ineradicable part of [our] society and culture."[1] The task at hand is not to solve a problem once and for all, but to continuously manage a perennially challenging social predicament. In a nation of some 240 million people, any measure that influences the drinking behavior of even 1 percent of teenagers or adults will each year save thousands of lives and prevent countless episodes of alcohol-related personal, medical, and social distress.

The progress that our nation has made in the past twenty years in reducing cigarette smoking can serve as an inspiring example of the combined overall effect of many measures, each of which may seem relatively limited. The percentage of the population that smokes has significantly declined, in part because many smokers have quit and in part because fewer nonsmokers are taking up smoking. Contributing factors to this cheering result include:

adverse publicity generated by the Surgeon General's reports

prohibition of cigarette advertising on television and radio mandatory health warnings on each package of cigarettes and in each print ad or billboard

increases in price and in taxes on cigarettes

increase in public service advertising against smoking

dissemination of new research on the health risks of smoking, particularly for pregnant women and people who have ailments such as high blood pressure or heart disease

dissemination of new research on the hazards of secondary smoke to nonsmokers and subsequent redefinition of smokers' and nonsmokers' rights in the workplace and in other public places.

Similarly, we have seen broad national changes in other health-related daily activities. On the average we are eating less beef and more fish, fewer eggs and more grains; and more of us are exercising more regularly than Americans did thirty years ago.

## Drinking as an Influenceable Behavior

The overall theme that must guide social policies on heavy drinking is that we are not dealing with an illness but with an activity that—like bad diet, lack of exercise, or smoking—tends to cause illness. The main line of attack must focus on the imprudent forms of behavior that become importantly enmeshed in a person's way of life and that may later lead to illness. If we can prevent or reduce the harmful behavior, the medical problems will never arise.

Studies sponsored by the National Research Council have pioneered the domain of large-scale, mass-oriented measures to manage our nation's alcohol problems. As one of these reports argued, "The possibilities for reducing the [alcohol] problem by preventive measures are modest but real and should increase with experience; they should not be ignored because of ghosts from the past."² (Surely, one of these ghosts is the classic disease concept, with its emphasis on heavy drinking as a medical problem.) Although experts still disagree about which techniques are the most promising, support for the measures described in this chapter is wide enough to warrant their serious consideration.³

One cluster of techniques is aimed at reducing the availability of alcohol. No one is proposing that we reenact Prohibition—although during its tenure alcohol consumption and the incidence of alcohol-related illness declined. The issue, rather, is whether alcohol should be as conveniently and cheaply available as it now is in many states. Might increasing liquor taxes, reducing the number of stores licensed to sell beer and liquor, or mandating an earlier closing time for bars reduce alcohol abuse without interfering too much with the preferences and pleasures of social drinkers? Let's look at the evidence on the likely effects of specific measures.

State and federal liquor taxes, a key component of retail liquor prices, have not increased at anything like the rate of inflation since the 1950s. Thus the real cost of liquor has dropped. As a number of studies have shown, a decrease in the real cost of alcohol tends to be followed by a rise in consumption levels; and an increase in the real cost tends to lower consumption levels. Moreover, moderate changes in cost affect consumption throughout the drinking population, including long-term heavy drinkers.⁴

Calculations based on prices in 1981 tell us, for example, that an increase of sixteen cents in the cost of a fifth of liquor would reduce liver cirrhosis mortality by 1.9 percent—or, since about 30,000 people in the U.S. die from this liver disease each year—by about 600 deaths. On this same basis, doubling the federal liquor tax from $1.68 per fifth of liquor to $3.36 would decrease cirrhosis mortality by about 6,000 cases each year. And we should note that had the federal liquor tax kept up with inflation since 1951, today the tax would be about $5.00 per fifth of liquor.[5]

Of course, even among the heaviest drinkers, only a minority die of liver cirrhosis. But at least one researcher affirms that "it is a reasonable assumption that changes in cirrhosis mortality reflect changes in all those problems that result from the chronic heavy use of alcohol."[6] If indeed this is true, a decline in cirrhosis would be a bellwether of declines in other alcohol-associated illnesses, accidents, and deaths. Furthermore, any drop in consumption by drinkers who are not long-term heavy drinkers would also yield positive benefits, especially since this group is far larger than the chronic alcohol-abusing population.

Most unfortunately for the purposes of public understanding, deaths or accidents that are prevented by sound public policy are measured in statistics that cannot be filmed for TV, that do not appear on hospital records or police blotters, and are not the subjects of news stories. There is no easy way to dramatize the great human suffering and family tragedies that do not take place but would have had it not been for an increase in the price of alcohol. And while our intuition may tell us that sixteen or sixty cents can't make much difference, minimal price increases do produce real effects.

Other aspects of alcohol availability also seem to influence consumption. A case in point: When legal restrictions on liquor purchases were greatly liberalized in Finland in the 1960s, alcoholic beverage consumption rapidly doubled. While other influences were at work as well, there was a significant causal relation between the liberalized availability and the rise in consumption.[7]

The number and diversity of retail alcohol outlets is governed by state licensing, and states could take it upon themselves to experiment with limits on the number and location of distribution outlets and their hours of service. In turn, the demand for licenses is influenced by the profitability of liquor sales, and steps could be taken to modestly reduce profitability—enough to make a marginal difference—without being oppressive or confiscatory.[8] The goal of such measures should not be to massively curtail liquor sales, only to provide a bit of added inconvenience that might marginally discourage purchases.

Legitimate questions have been raised by experts about the adequacy of the evidence for these approaches.[9] But measures to control the availability of alcohol are at least worthy of a public hearing and, if nothing else, they can turn the course of public debate toward the notion that modest measures—rather than grand sweeping solutions—are the best tools we have.

Of course, the liquor interests generally oppose any regulations aimed at reducing overall levels of consumption, and even the most modest proposals on pricing or licensing will elicit intense lobbying. The fate of any effort to pare liquor sales will therefore require a broad political coalition convinced that minor adjustments in the liquor laws can achieve a positive marginal effect.

That such measures will only affect casual drinkers, that heavy drinkers are oblivious to price hikes or reduced availability, is a fallacious residue of the disease concept of alcoholism, a ghost from the past.

## Social Norms

The National Research Council study also recommends that broad educational, advertising, and public information campaigns be undertaken to change our society's drinking customs and attitudes. The alcoholic beverage industry spends $1 billion a year on advertising and receives what amounts to free advertising whenever television programs or movies show attractive people in attractive settings routinely drinking, often heavily, as an integral part of their activities. (On television the beverage most often consumed is distilled liquor, even though in real life only about 16 percent of the beverages drunk by Americans are alcoholic.) [10]

Recent public service advertising seems already to have had an effect on shaping opinion and attitudes. [11] In the past few years there has been a significant shift away from the harder liquors to low-alcohol and nonalcoholic beverages.

## Legal Liability and Social Responsibility

Other specific efforts have been aimed not so much at the drinker but at the server, the host at a private party and the bartender at the neighborhood pub. New programs for training those who serve liquor to the public, for example, are intended to give servers a new sensitivity to and sense of responsibility for their customers' drinking and subsequent behavior. [12]

Although refusing to serve a visibly intoxicated person may initially seem socially awkward or intrusive on the rights of drinkers, the extension of social and legal responsibility to private hosts and bartenders is only one more example of contemporary social expectations about the liabilities that fall to the providers of goods and services. In all areas, manufacturers and distributors are required to attend to product safety, which includes the design, manufacturing, and labeling of products, and they are required to warn buyers of potentially dangerous products about the hazards of misuse. Of course, the individual drinker must be held to account for irresponsible conduct, but others who negligently contribute to that irresponsible conduct can no longer consider themselves blameless.

Increasingly, the courts are therefore holding bars and restaurants liable for damage committed by patrons who drank excessively and then caused harm while drunk. Recognizing that no one can be infallible in judging when to refuse service, state legislatures are moving to protect bartenders who complete server's intervention training from legal liability.

Changing attitudes and customs are also encouraging private hosts to assume some responsibility—moral, if not legal—in serving alcohol to their guests. Again, the goal is not to preach abstention, but to curtail excessive drinking. Hosts need not hover over guests, but neither should they feel that ignoring obvious intoxication is correct etiquette or socially gracious behavior.

## Protective Measures

Another set of social policies is intended to minimize the harms associated with heavy drinking. The core strategy resembles our approach to traffic safety. Even though we encourage every driver to be careful, a certain number will on occasion drive recklessly. We hold these drivers responsible for any harm they cause, but we also take practical measures to prevent or minimize the damage. We know that traffic lights at dangerous intersections are more effective than signs urging people to drive more carefully; that road bumps are more effective than posting a speed limit of five miles an hour; and that freeway median barriers are more effective than double yellow lines in preventing head-on collisions. We also press for better safety features in the automobiles we drive and stronger enforcement of traffic laws.

In sum, we try to prevent negligence and recklessness but also to minimize the damage to the innocent, and even to the guilty, from the accidents that do occur. Along this line, we could reduce the carnage associated with excessive drinking by demanding more research on simple and cheap devices to prevent the operation of dangerous machinery—automobiles, trucks, cranes, trains, buses—by anyone who falls below a certain level of muscular and mental coordination due to intoxication.[13] At least four states now require ignition-lock devices on the cars of convicted drinking-driver offenders to prevent the car from being started by a driver who fails to pass a breathalyzer test. Evaluation of the long-term practical efficacy of such devices in forestalling drinking and driving remains to be done, but even a 10 percent reduction would be considered a success by the authorities.[14] The proper question is not whether these devices are foolproof, but whether they produce some significant results, however modest, that prevent some traffic fatalities and injuries.

The costs of these protective measures have to be related to the moral and financial costs of the accidents that would otherwise have occurred. But just as insurance reimburses the victims of carelessness instead of relying solely on the careless offender to pay, social measures can be adopted to reduce harms caused by careless or reckless drinkers.[15]

## Conclusions

I could continue to list all the important social strategies intended to reduce alcohol abuse in this country: increasing traffic penalties for drunk driving, instituting random road checks, enforcing the prohibition of sales to minors, rewriting the regulations governing advertising, and a host of other approaches. But this is not a book about the entirety of alcohol use and abuse in modern America.

Rather, my aim has been limited to calling to the reader's attention the scientific evidence that disproves the classic disease concept of alcoholism and encourages an alternative perspective: seeing heavy drinking as a meaningful part of a drinker's way of life. Once we leave behind the disease concept, which emphasizes medicine and individual treatment for a supposedly involuntary symptom, we can adopt a broader view: that what takes place in the drinker's environment may be more important than what takes place in the drinker's body.

Thus in this chapter I have not attempted to present a complete inventory of social experiments. But I trust that I have offered enough empirical evidence and authoritative opinions to establish the principle that social strategies can have an effect even on so-called addicted drinkers, as well as a salutary influence on potential heavy drinkers. Just as we hope that troubled individual drinkers can reshape their ways of life, so too can we as a society begin to reshape our attitudes, beliefs, and behaviors concerning alcohol abuse.

## Notes

1. M. Moore and Gerstein, *Alcohol and Public Policy* (1981), 116. See also Mäkela, "Lessons from the Postwar Period" (1985), 19.
2. Olson and Gerstein, *Alcohol in America* (1985), v. The National Research Council is the principal research agency of the National Academy of Sciences and the National Institute of Medicine, the federal government's most prestigious scientific organizations.
3. See Bruun et al., *Alcohol Control Policies* (1975); WHO Expert Committee on Problems Related to Alcohol Consumption, *Problems Related to Alcohol Consumption* (1980); Gerstein, *Toward the Prevention of Alcohol Problems* (1984); M. Moore and Gerstein (1981). Two collections of relevant studies are Grant, *Economics and Alcohol* (1983), and Grant, *Alcohol Policies* (1985).
4. Olson and Gerstein (1985), chap. 4; P. Cook, "Increasing the Federal Alcohol Excise Tax" (1984); P. Cook, "The Effect of Liquor Taxes on Drinking, Cirrhosis, and Auto Accidents" (1981); Mäkela et al., *Alcohol, Society, and the State* (1981), 90; Schmidt, "Cirrhosis and Alcohol Consumption" (1976).

   Much of the line of thought about social control of consumption and its effect on the entire spectrum of drinkers derives from

Ledermann, *Alcool, Alcoolisme, Alcoolisation*, I and II (1956; 1964). For representative criticism of this approach, see Pittman, "An Evaluation of the Control of Consumption Policy" (1983). For challenges to the effect of taxation, see Walsh, "The Economics of Alcohol Taxation" (1983).

5. Olson and Gerstein (1985), 45, 52–53; see also P. Cook (1984), 28.

6. Schmidt (1976), 15–16. See also Mäkela et al. (1981), 90.

7. Olson and Gerstein (1985), 59–60; Beauchamp, *Beyond Alcoholism* (1980), 144.

8. The relationships between regulation and consumption are still a matter of study and debate; in some situations consumption may decline after regulations are relaxed; see M. Moore and Gerstein (1981), 78. The classic work on this subject is Bruun et al. (1975). See also Clayson, "The Role of Licensing Law in Limiting the Misuse of Alcohol" (1976); and Mäkela et al. (1981).

9. For example, Stanton Peele and Robin Room have debated the issues in a series of articles; see Peele "The Limitations of Control-of-Supply Models for Explaining and Preventing Alcoholism and Drug Addiction" (1987a); Room "Alcohol Control, Addiction, and Processes of Change" (1987); and Peele, "What Does Addiction Have to Do with Level of Consumption?" (1987b). See also the economic analyses by the contributors to Grant (1983).

10. Data in this paragraph are from Olson and Gerstein (1985), 82–84. See also "Alcohol: Advertising, Counteradvertising, and Depiction in the Public Media" (1986), 1486.

11. See Grant (1985), 143–47.

12. Olson and Gerstein (1985), chaps. 4 and 5; Knobeldorff, "Programs Provide Roadblock to Drunk-Driving" (1986); Gerstein (1984), 57–67.

13. Olson and Gerstein (1985), 43, describe several ignition devices that test an operator's level of intoxication.

14. Sullivan, "New Device Takes Ignition Keys Out of the Hands of Drinking Drivers" (1987); A. Cook, "A New Push on Drunken Drivers" (1987).

15. For detailed discussion of other social measures, see Moser, *Prevention of Alcohol-Related Problems* (1980); Olson and Gerstein (1985); Gerstein (1984); M. Moore and Gerstein (1981); WHO Expert Committee (1980).

# AFTERWORD

I wrote this book out of a sense of urgency, believing it was imperative to inform the general public of the latest research on heavy drinking and of the sea change that has occurred in professional scientific circles. Because I knew that outdated and often false ideas were firmly rooted in most people's minds, I felt that this was not an occasion for pussyfooting around the evidence nor for presenting a numbingly detailed analysis of every bit of the evidence. But I have tried to use the sources responsibly and fairly, if somewhat confrontationally, to illuminate the central issues that ought to concern the general public.

As we have seen, scientists are far from agreeing on an explanation of why some people become heavy drinkers, and there is no unanimity about how best to help chronic heavy drinkers. But whatever specific views seem most persuasive to you about the causes or treatment of heavy drinking, there are some broad premises and conclusions we all must accept. Clearly, we can never hope to prevent all alcohol abuse in our society. Social drinking is pervasive in our history and culture, and every social activity is subject to abuse. Nor should

144

we expect that anyone will develop a therapeutic regimen that will help every heavy drinker change his or her way of life.

Yet we need not throw up our hands in despair. Although we must surrender all utopian dreams of a technological breakthrough that will make the problem disappear, we can take heart in several of the findings reported in this book. First, to some degree the problems of heavy drinkers are self-limiting; that is, many heavy drinkers, without any formal intervention, do return to moderate drinking or abstinence. Second, researchers are continuing to learn more about ways to help heavy drinkers who do seek assistance. Third, we have recently seen a healthy increase in local and national experimentation with social policies designed to discourage excessive drinking.

I suspect that many of you know someone who is a heavy drinker or a problem drinker and that you are wondering what can be done to help that person. At this time, there are no simple answers. Heavy drinkers can and do learn to change their ways of life—and far more often than the advertisements for disease-oriented treatment centers would have us believe. But there is no guaranteed technique, no magic formula that will prompt or produce this change.

I know that this answer is not the one most people want to hear. Yet rather than succumbing to the promises of the latest fad, we need to be candid about our knowledge and our ignorance. I hope that in this book I have made a start in that direction by debunking some of the myths and mistruths that have so long dominated the discussion of heavy drinking.

# WORKS CITED

Adesso, Vincent J. 1985. "Cognitive Factors in Alcohol and Drug Use." In Galizio and Maisto (1985), 179–208.

"Alcohol: Advertising, Counteradvertising, and Depiction in the Public Media." 1986. *JAMA, Journal of the American Medical Association* 256:1485–88.

*Alcohol: Use and Abuse in America.* 1985. Gallup Report no. 242. Princeton: The Gallup Report.

*Alcohol and Alcoholism.* 1979. Report of a Special Committee of the Royal College of Psychiatrists. London: Tavistock.

*Alcohol and Health.* 1971. First special report to the Congress. Washington, D.C.: Department of Health, Education and Welfare.

*Alcoholics Anonymous.* 1955. New York: A.A. World Services.

American Medical Association. 1967. *Manual on Alcoholism.*

Armor, David J. 1980. "The RAND Reports and the Analysis of Relapse." In Edwards and Grant (1980), 81–94.

Armor, David J.; Polich, J. Michael; and Stambul, Harriet B. 1976. *Alcoholism and Treatment.* Santa Monica, Calif.: The Rand Corporation.

Austin, Gregory A., and Prendergast, Michael L. 1987. "Chronology of Alcohol Use and Controls: Europe from Antiquity to 1800." In Barrows, Room, and Verhay (1987), 189.

Baeklund, F.; Lundwall, L.; and Kissin, B. 1975. "Methods for the Treatment of Chronic Alcoholism: A Critical Approach." In R. J.

Gibbons, Y. Israel, H. Kalant, R. E. Popham, and R. G. Smart, eds., *Research Advances in Alcohol and Drug Problems*, 2:247–327. New York: Wiley.

Barr, Harriet L.; Ottenberg, Donald J.; Antes, Derry; and Rosen, Alvin. 1984. "Mortality of Treated Alcoholics and Drug Addicts: The Benefits of Abstinence." *Journal of Studies on Alcohol* 45: 440–52.

Barrows, Susan; Room, Robin; and Verhay, Jeffrey, eds. 1987. *The Social History of Alcohol*. Berkeley, Calif.: Alcohol Research Group.

Beauchamp, Dan E. 1980. *Beyond Alcoholism*. Philadelphia: Temple University Press.

Bernard, Joel. 1984. "From the Fast Day Sermon to the Temperance Address: The Psychic Origins of a Social Movement." Conference on the Social History of Alcohol, Berkeley, Calif.

Biernacki, Patrick. 1986. *Pathways from Heroin Addiction: Recovery Without Treatment*. Philadelphia: Temple University Press.

Bigelow, W., and Liebson, I. 1972. "Cost Factors Controlling Alcoholic Drinking." *Psychological Record* 22:305–14.

Blane, H. T. 1968. *The Personality of the Alcoholic*. New York: Harper & Row.

Boffey, Philip M. 1982. "Alcoholism Study Under New Attack." *New York Times*, June 28.

Bohman, M.; Sigvardsson, S.; and Cloninger, C. R. 1981. "Maternal Inheritance of Alcohol Abuse." *Archives of General Psychiatry* 38: 965–69.

Brewer, W. F. 1974. "There Is No Convincing Evidence for Operant or Classical Conditioning in Adult Humans." In W. B. Weiner and D. J. Palermo, eds., *Cognition and the Symbolic Processes*, 1–42. Hillsdale, N.J.: Lawrence Erlbaum Associates.

Brickman, P.; Rabinowitz, V. C.; Karuza, J.; Coates, D.; Cohn, E.; and Kidder, L. 1982. "Models of Helping and Coping." *American Psychologist* 37:368–84.

Brownell, Kelly D.; Marlatt, G. Alan; Lichtenstein, Edward; and Wilson, G. Terence. 1986. "Understanding and Preventing Relapse." *American Psychologist* 41:765–82.

Brunner-Orne, M. 1963. "Comment on 'Normal' Drinking in Recovered Alcohol Addicts." *Quarterly Journal of Studies on Alcohol* 24:730–33.

Bruun, Kettil; Edwards, G.; Lumio, M.; Mäkela, K.; and others. 1975. *Alcohol Control Policies in Public Health Perspective*. Forssa, Finland: Finnish Foundation for Alcohol Studies.

Caddy, Glenn R. 1978. "Towards a Multivariate Analysis of Alcohol Abuse." In Nathan, Marlatt, and Loberg (1978), 71–117.

———. 1982. "A Multivariate Approach to Restricted Drinking." In William M. Hay and Peter E. Nathan, eds., *Clinical Case Studies in the Behavioral Treatment of Alcoholism*, 275–96. New York: Plenum Press.

Caddy, Glenn R., and Block, Trudy. 1985. "Individual Differences in Response to Treatment." In Galizio and Maisto (1985), 317–62.

Cadoret, R., and Gath, A. 1978. "Inheritance of Alcoholism in Adoptees." *British Journal of Psychiatry* 132:252–58.

Caetano, Raul. 1987. "Public Opinions About Alcoholism and Its Treatment." *Journal of Alcohol Studies* 48:153–60.

Cahalan, Don. 1978. "Subcultural Differences in Drinking Behavior in U.S. National Surveys and Selected European Studies." In Nathan, Marlatt, and Loberg (1978), 235–53.

Cahalan, Don, and Room, Robin. 1974. *Problem Drinking Among American Men*. New Brunswick, N.J.: Rutgers Center of Alcohol Studies.

Canter, F. M. 1968. "The Requirement of Abstinence as a Problem in Institutional Treatment of Alcoholics." *Psychiatric Quarterly* 42:217–31.

Cappell, H., and LeBlanc, A. E. 1981. "Tolerance and Physical Dependence: Do They Play a Role in Alcohol and Drug Self-Administration?" In Israel et al. (1981), 159–96.

Clare, Anthony. 1976. "How Good Is Treatment?" In Edwards and Grant (1976), 279–89.

Clark, W. B. 1975. "Conceptions of Alcoholism: Consequences for Research." *Addictive Diseases* 1:395.

Clark, W. B., and Cahalan, D. 1976. "Changes in Problem Drinking over a Four-Year Span." *Addictive Behaviors* 1:251–59.

Clayson, C. 1976. "The Role of Licensing Law in Limiting the Misuse of Alcohol." In Edwards and Grant (1976), 78–87.

Cloninger, C. R.; Bohman, M.; and Sigvardsson, S. 1981. "Inheritance of Alcohol Abuse: Cross-Fostering Analysis of Adopted Men." *Archives of General Psychiatry* 38:861–68.

Cohen, M.; Liebson, I.; Fallace, L.; and Speers, W. 1971a. "Alcoholism: Controlled Drinking and Incentives for Abstinence." *Psychological Reports* 28:575–80.

Cohen, M.; Liebson, I.; Fallace, L.; and Allen, R. 1971b. "Moderate Drinking by Chronic Alcoholics: A Schedule-Dependent Phenomenon." *Journal of Nervous and Mental Disease* 153:434–44.

Cook, Alberta I. 1987. "A New Push on Drunken Drivers." *The National Law Journal*, Feb. 9, pp. 3, 8.

Cook, Philip J. 1981. "The Effect of Liquor Taxes on Drinking, Cirrhosis, and Auto Accidents." In M. Moore and Gerstein (1981), 255–85.

———. 1984. "Increasing the Federal Alcohol Excise Tax." In Gerstein (1984), 24–32.

Costello, Raymond M. 1980. "Alcoholism Treatment Effectiveness: Slicing the Outcome Variance Pie." In Edwards and Grant (1980), 113–27.

Cox, W. Miles. 1985. "Personality Correlates of Substance Abuse." In Galizio and Maisto (1985), 209–46.

Crawford, Alex. 1987. "Attitudes About Alcohol: A General Review." *Drug and Alcohol Dependence* 19:279.

Davies, D. L. 1962. "Normal Drinking in Recovered Alcohol Addicts." *Quarterly Journal of Studies on Alcohol* 23:94–104.

Davies, Phil. 1985. "Does Treatment Work? A Sociological Perspective." In Heather, Robertson, and Davies (1985), 158–77.

Deitrich, Richard A., and Spuhler, Karen. 1984. "Genetics of Alcoholism and Alcohol Actions." In Smart et al. (1984), 47–98.

Donovan, D. M., and Marlatt, G. A. 1980. "Assessment of Expectancies and Behavior Associated with Alcohol Consumption: A Cognitive-Behavioral Approach." *Journal of Studies on Alcohol* 41:1153–85.

Edwards, Griffith. 1970. "The Status of Alcoholism as a Disease." In R. V. Phillipson, ed., *Modern Trends in Drug Dependence and Alcoholism*, 1:119–63. London: Butterworths.

———. 1976. "The Alcohol Dependence Syndrome: Usefulness of an Idea." In Edwards and Grant (1976), 136–56.

———. 1985. "A Later Follow-up of a Classic Case Series: D. L. Davies's 1962 Report and Its Significance for the Present." *Journal of Studies on Alcohol* 46:181–90.

Edwards, Griffith, and Grant, Marcus. 1976. *Alcoholism: New Knowledge and New Responses*. Baltimore: University Park Press.

———, eds. 1980. *Alcoholism Treatment in Transition*. Baltimore: University Park Press.

Edwards, Griffith; Hensman, C.; Hawker, A.; Williamson, V. 1967. "Alcoholics Anonymous: The Anatomy of a Self-Help Group." *Social Psychiatry* 1:4.

Edwards, Griffith; Gross, Milton M.; Keller, Mark; Moser, Joy; and Room, Robin, eds. 1977. *Alcohol-Related Disabilities*. WHO Offset Publication no. 32. Geneva: World Health Organization.

Edwards, Griffith; Bewley, T. H.; Connell, P. H.; Glatt, M. M.; Milne, H. B.; Murray, R. M.; Oppenheim, A. N.; and Walton, H. J. 1979. *Alcohol and Alcoholism.* Report of a Special Committee of the Royal College of Psychiatrists. London: Tavistock.

Engle, K. B., and Williams, T. K. 1972. "Effect of an Ounce of Vodka on Alcoholics' Desire for Alcohol." *Quarterly Journal of Studies on Alcohol* 33:1099–1105.

Ewing, J. A., and Rouse, B. A. 1976. "Failure of an Experimental Treatment Programme to Inculcate Controlled Drinking in Alcoholics." *British Journal of Addiction* 71:123–34.

Fingarette, Herbert. 1970. "The Perils of Powell: In Search of a Factual Foundation for the 'Disease Concept of Alcoholism.'" *Harvard Law Review* 83:793–812.

———. 1975. "Addiction and Criminal Responsibility." *Yale Law Journal* 84:413–46.

———. 1979. "How an Alcoholism Defense Works Under the ALI Insanity Test." *International Journal of Law and Psychiatry* 2:299–322.

———. 1981. "Legal Aspects of Alcoholism and Other Addictions: Some Basic Conceptual Issues." *British Journal of Addiction* 76:125–32.

———. 1983. "Philosophical and Legal Aspects of the Disease Concept of Alcoholism." In Smart et al. (1983), 1–46.

———. 1984. "Excuse: Intoxication." In Sanford Kadish, ed., *Encyclopedia of Criminal Justice.* New York: Free Press.

———. 1985a. "Alcoholism: Neither Sin nor Disease." *The Center Magazine* 18(3): 56–63.

———. 1985b. "Alcoholism and Self-Deception." In M. W. Martin, ed., *Self-Deception and Self-Understanding.* Lawrence: University of Kansas Press.

Fingarette, Herbert, and Hasse, Ann F. 1979. *Mental Disabilities and Criminal Responsibility.* Berkeley: University of California Press.

Franks, Lucinda. 1985. "A New Attack on Alcoholism." *New York Times Magazine,* Oct. 20.

Frawley, P. Joseph. 1987. "Neurobehavioral Model of Addiction." *Journal of Drug Issues* 17:29–46.

Fuller, R. K., and Roth, H. P. 1979. "Disulfiram for the Treatment of Alcoholism: An Evaluation in 128 Men." *Annals of Internal Medicine* 90:901–4.

Fuller, R. K., and Williford, W. O. 1980. "Life-table Analysis of Abstinence in a Study Evaluating the Efficacy of Disulfiram." *Alcoholism: Clinical and Experimental Research* 4:298–301.

Fuller, R. K.; Branchey, L.; Brightwell, D.; Derman, R.; and others. 1986. "Disulfiram Treatment of Alcoholism: A Veterans Administration Cooperative Study." *JAMA, Journal of the American Medical Association* 256:1449–55.

Galizio, Mark, and Maisto, Stephen A. 1985. *Determinants of Substance Abuse: Biological, Psychological, and Environmental Factors.* New York: Plenum Press.

Gerard, D. L.; Sanger, G.; and Wile, R. 1962. "The Abstinent Alcoholic." *Archives of General Psychiatry* 6:99–111.

Gerstein, Dean R. 1984. *Toward the Prevention of Alcohol Problems.* Washington, D.C.: National Academy Press.

Glaser, Frederick B. 1980. "Anybody Got a Match? Treatment Research and the Matching Hypothesis." In Edwards and Grant (1980), 178–96.

Glaser, Frederick B., and Skinner, Harvey A. 1981. "Matching in the Real World: A Practical Approach." In Gottheil, McLellan, and Druley (1981), 295–324.

Glatt, M. M. 1976. "Alcoholism Disease Concept and Loss of Control Revisited." *British Journal of Addiction* 71:135.

———. 1982. "The 'Lack of Control' over Alcohol and Its Implications." In M. M. Glatt and J. Marks, *The Dependence Phenomenon,* 119–55. Ridgewood, N.J.: Bogden & Son.

Goodwin, Donald W. 1985. "Genetic Determinants of Alcoholism." In Mendelson and Mello (1985), 65–87.

Goodwin, Donald W.; Schulsinger, F.; Hermansen, L.; Guze, S. B.; and Winokur, G. 1973. "Alcohol Problems in Adoptees Raised Apart from Alcoholic Biological Parents." *Archives of General Psychiatry* 28:238–43.

Gottheil, Edward; McLellan, A. Thomas; and Druley, Keith A. 1981. *Matching Patient Needs and Treatment Methods in Alcoholism and Drug Abuse.* Springfield, Ill.: Charles C. Thomas.

Gottheil, Edward; Corbett, Lacey O.; Grassburger, Joseph C.; and Cornelison, Floyd S. 1972. "Fixed Interval Drinking Decisions, I: A Research and Treatment Model." *Quarterly Journal of Studies on Alcohol* 33:311–24.

Gottheil, Edward; Alterman, A.; Skoloda, T. E.; and Murphy, B. F. 1973. "Alcoholics' Patterns of Controlled Drinking." *American Journal of Psychiatry* 130:418–22.

Grant, Marcus, ed. 1983. *Economics and Alcohol.* New York: Gardner Press.

———, ed. 1985. *Alcohol Policies.* World Health Organization, Regional Publications, European series, no. 18.

Gusfield, Joseph R. 1963. *Symbolic Crusade: Status Politics and the American Temperance Movement*. Urbana: University of Illinois Press.

———. 1981. *The Culture of Public Problems: Drinking-Driving and the Symbolic Order*. Chicago: University of Chicago Press.

Heather, Nick, and Robertson, Ian. 1981. *Controlled Drinking*. London: Methuen.

Heather, Nick; Robertson, Ian; and Davies, Phil, eds. 1985. *The Misuse of Alcohol*. New York: New York University Press.

Hill, Thomas W. 1987. "Alcohol Use Among the Nebraska Winnebago: An Ethnohistorical Study of Change and Adjustment." In Barrows, Room, and Verhay (1987), 106.

Hingson, Ralph; Scotch, Norman; and Goldman, Eli. 1977. "Impact of the 'Rand Report' on Alcoholics, Treatment Personnel and Boston Residents." *Journal of Studies on Alcohol* 38:2065–86.

Hodgson, Ray. 1976. "Behaviour Therapy." In Edwards and Grant (1976), 290–307.

Hodgson, Ray; Rankin, Howard; and Stockwell, Tim. 1978. "Craving and Loss of Control." In Nathan, Marlatt, and Loberg (1978), 341–49.

———. 1979. "Alcohol Dependence and the Priming Effect." *Behaviour Research and Therapy* 17:379–87.

Holden, Constance. 1987a. "Alcoholism and the Medical Cost Crunch." *Science* 235:1132–33.

———. 1987b. "Is Alcoholism Treatment Effective?" *Science* 236: 20–22.

Hore, Brian D. 1976. *Alcohol Dependence*. London: Butterworths.

Hunt, G. P. 1987. "Spirits of the Colonial Economy." In Barrows, Room, and Verhay (1987), 269.

Israel, Y.; Glaser, Frederick; Kalant, Harold; Popham, Robert; Schmidt, Wolfgang; Smart, Raymond, eds. 1978. *Research Advances in Alcohol and Drug Problems*, vol. 4. New York: Plenum Press.

———, eds. 1981. *Research Advances in Alcohol and Drug Problems*, vol. 6. New York: Plenum Press.

Jaffe, Jerome H., and Ciraulo, Domenic A. 1985. "Drugs Used in the Treatment of Alcoholism." In Mendelson and Mello (1985), 355–89.

Jellinek, E. M. 1946. "Phases in the Drinking History of Alcoholics." *Quarterly Journal of Studies on Alcohol* 7:1–88.

———. 1952. "The Phases of Alcohol Addiction." *Quarterly Journal of Studies on Alcohol* 13:673–84.

────. 1960. *The Disease Concept of Alcoholism*. New Haven, Conn.: Hillhouse Press.

Kaij, L. 1960. *Alcoholism in Twins*. Stockholm: Almquest & Wilsell.

Kaplan, John. 1983. *The Hardest Drug: Heroin and Public Policy*. Chicago: University of Chicago Press.

Keller, Mark. 1972. "On the Loss-of-Control Phenomenon in Alcoholism." *British Journal of Addiction* 67:153–66.

────. 1978. "A Nonbehaviorist's View of the Behavioral Problem with Alcoholism." In Nathan, Marlatt, and Loberg (1978), 381–97.

Kissin, Benjamin. 1977. "Alcoholism: A Controlled Trial of 'Treatment' and 'Advice'" [comments]. *Journal of Studies on Alcohol* 38:1804–8.

────. 1983. "The Disease Concept of Alcoholism." In Smart et al. (1983), 93–126.

Knobeldorff, Kerry E. 1986. "Programs Provide Roadblock to Drunk-Driving." *Christian Science Monitor*, Aug. 28.

LaPorte, D. J.; McLellan, A. T.; Erdlen, F. R.; and Parente, R. J. 1981. "Treatment Outcome as a Function of Follow-up Difficulty in Substance Abusers." *Journal of Consulting and Clinical Psychology* 49:112–19.

Ledermann, S. 1956. *Alcool, Alcoolisme, Alcoolisation*, I. Paris: Presses Universitaires de France.

────. 1964. *Alcool, Alcoolisme, Alcoolisation*, II. Paris: Presses Universitaires de France.

Lemere, F., and Voegtlin, W. L. 1950. "An Evaluation of the Aversion Treatment of Alcoholism." *Quarterly Journal of Studies on Alcohol* 11:199–204.

Lenke, Leif. 1984. "Total Consumption of Alcohol and 'Heavy Use': The Swedish Case." *Surveyor*, no. 19, p. 53.

Levine, Harry G. 1978. "The Discovery of Addiction: Changing Conceptions of Habitual Drunkenness in America." *Journal of Studies on Alcohol* 39:143–74.

────. 1981. "The Good Creature of God and the Demon Rum: Colonial America and 19th-Century Ideas About Alcohol, Crime, and Accidents." In Room and Collins (1981), 111–85.

Lindros, Kai O. 1978. "Acetaldehyde—Its Metabolism and Role in the Action of Alcohol." In Israel et al. (1978), 111–76.

Ludwig, A.; Wikler, A.; and Stark, L. H. 1974. "The First Drink: Psychobiological Aspects of Craving." *Archives of General Psychiatry* 30:539–47.

MacAndrew, C., and Edgerton, R. B. 1969. *Drunken Comportment*. Chicago: Aldine.

McClelland, D. C.; Davis, W. N.; Kalin, R.; and Wanner, E. 1972. *The Drinking Man.* New York: Free Press.

McLachlan, John F. C. 1974. "Therapy Strategies, Personality Orientation, and Recovery from Alcoholism." *Canadian Psychiatric Association Journal* 19:25–30.

Maisto, Stephen A.; Galizio, Mark; and Carey, Kate B. 1985. "Individual Differences in Substance Abuse." In Galizio and Maisto (1985), 3–12.

Maisto, Stephen A.; Lauerman, R.; and Adesso, V. J. 1977. "A Comparison of Two Experimental Studies Investigating the Role of Cognitive Factors in Excessive Drinking." *Journal of Studies on Alcohol* 38:145–49.

Mäkela, K. 1980. "What Can Medicine Properly Take On?" In Edwards and Grant (1980), 225–33.

————. 1985. "Lessons from the Postwar Period." In Grant and Marcus (1985), 9–22.

Mäkela, K.; Room, R.; Single, E.; Sulkunen, P.; Walsh, B.; and others. 1981. *Alcohol, Society and the State: A Comparative Study of Alcohol Control,* vol. 1. Toronto: Addiction Research Foundation.

Mann, Marty. 1950. *Primer on Alcoholism.* New York: Rinehart.

Marlatt, G. Alan. 1978. "Craving for Alcohol, Loss of Control, and Relapse: A Cognitive-Behavioral Analysis." In Nathan, Marlatt, and Loberg (1978), 271–314.

————. 1982. "Psychosocial Perspectives on Alcoholism Treatment and the Process of Recovery." Conference on Directions in Alcohol Abuse Treatment Research. Newport, R.I.

————. 1983. "The Controlled Drinking Controversy." *American Psychologist* 38:1097–1110.

————. 1985. "Relapse Prevention: Theoretical Rationale and Overview of the Model." In Marlatt and Gordon (1985), 3–70.

Marlatt, G. Alan; Deming, B.; and Reid, J. B. 1973. "Loss of Control Drinking in Alcoholics: An Experimental Analogue." *Journal of Abnormal Psychology* 81:233–41.

Marlatt, G. Alan, and Donovan, D. M. 1982. "Behavioral Psychology Approaches to Alcoholism." In E. M. Pattison and E. Kaufman, eds., *Encyclopedic Handbook of Alcoholism.* New York: Gardner Press.

Marlatt, G. Alan, and Gordon, Judith, eds. 1985. *Relapse Prevention.* New York: Guilford Press.

Marlatt, G. Alan, and Rohsenow, D. J. 1980. "Cognitive Processes in Alcohol Use: Expectancy and the Balanced Placebo Design." In

N. K. Mello, ed., *Advances in Substance Abuse: Behavioral and Biological Research*, vol. 1. Greenwich, Conn.: JAI Press.

Marshall, Mac. 1981. "'Four Hundred Rabbits': An Anthropological View of Ethanol as a Disinhibitor." In Room and Collins (1981), 186–204.

Mello, Nancy K. 1975. "A Semantic Aspect of Alcoholism." In H. Cappell and A. E. LeBlanc, eds., *Biological and Behavioural Approaches to Drug Dependence*, 73–87. Toronto: Addiction Research Foundation.

Mello, Nancy K., and Mendelson, J. H. 1970. "Experimentally Induced Intoxication in Alcoholics: A Comparison Between Programmed and Spontaneous Drinking." *Journal of Pharmacology and Experimental Therapeutics* 173:101–16.

———. 1972. "Drinking Patterns During Work-contingent and Non-contingent Alcohol Acquisition." *Psychosomatic Medicine* 34: 139–64.

———. 1985. *Alcohol: Use and Abuse in America*. Boston: Little, Brown.

Mendelson, Jack H., ed. 1964. "Experimentally Induced Chronic Intoxication and Withdrawal in Alcoholics." *Quarterly Journal of Studies on Alcohol*, supplement no. 2.

Mendelson, Jack H., and Mello, Nancy K. 1979. "One Unanswered Question About Alcoholism." *British Journal of Addiction* 74:11–14.

———. 1985. *The Diagnosis and Treatment of Alcoholism*. New York: McGraw Hill.

Mendelson, Jack H.; Babor, Thomas F.; Mello, Nancy K.; and Pratt, Herbert. 1986. "Alcoholism and Prevalence of Medical and Psychiatric Disorders." *Journal of Studies on Alcohol* 47:361.

Merry, J. 1966. "The 'Loss of Control' Myth." *Lancet* 1:1257–58.

Merry, J., and others. 1976. "Prophylactic Treatment of Alcoholism by Lithium Carbonate." *Lancet*, Sept. 4.

Miller, Peter M. 1976. *Behavioral Treatment of Alcoholism*. New York: Pergamon.

Miller, William R., and Hester, Reid K. 1986. "Inpatient Alcoholism Treatment: Who Benefits?" *American Psychologist* 41:794–805.

Moore, Mark H., and Gerstein, Dean R. 1981. *Alcohol and Public Policy*. Washington, D.C.: National Academy Press.

Moore, Robert A. 1985. "The Prevalence of Alcoholism in Medical and Surgical Patients." In Schuckit (1985c), 247–65.

Moser, Joy. 1980. *Prevention of Alcohol-Related Problems*. Toronto: World Health Organization, Alcoholism and Drug Addiction Research Foundation.

Nathan, Peter E., and Niaura, Raymond S. 1985. "Behavioral Assessment and Treatment of Alcoholism." In Mendelson and Mello (1985), 391–455.

Nathan, Peter E.; Marlatt, G. Alan; and Loberg, Tor, eds. 1978. *Alcoholism: New Directions in Behavioral Research and Treatment*. New York: Plenum Press.

National Council on Alcoholism. 1972. "Criteria for the Diagnosis of Alcoholism." *Annals of Internal Medicine* 77:249.

Neuberger, O. W.; Miller, S. I.; Schmitz, R. E.; Matarezzo, J. D.; Pratt, H.; and Hasha, N. 1982. "Replicable Abstinence Rates in an Alcoholism Treatment Program." *JAMA, Journal of the American Medical Association* 248:960–63.

Nordstrom, Goran, and Berglund, Mats. 1987. "A Prospective Study of Successful Long-Term Adjustment in Alcohol Dependence: Social Drinking Versus Abstinence." *Journal of Alcohol Studies* 48:95–103.

Ogborne, Alan C.; Sobell, Mark B.; and Sobell, Linda C. 1985. "The Significance of Environmental Factors for the Design and the Evaluation of Alcohol Treatment Programs." In Galizio and Maisto (1985), 363–82.

Olson, Steve, and Gerstein, Dean R. 1985. *Alcohol in America: Taking Action to Prevent Abuse*. Washington, D.C.: National Academy Press.

Orford, Jim. 1973. "A Comparison of Alcoholics Whose Drinking Is Totally Uncontrolled and Those Whose Drinking Is Mainly Controlled." *Behaviour Research and Therapy* 11:565–76.

———. 1976. "Alcoholism: What Psychology Offers." In Edwards and Grant (1976), 88–99.

———. 1985. *Excessive Appetites: A Psychological View of Addictions*. New York: Wiley.

Orford, Jim, and Edwards, Griffith. 1977. *Alcoholism—A Comparison of Treatment and Advice, with a Study of the Influence of Marriage*. Oxford: Oxford University Press.

Orford, Jim; Oppenheimer, E.; and Edwards, G. 1976. "Abstinence or Control: the Outcome for Excessive Drinkers Two Years After Consultation." *Behaviour Research and Therapy* 14:409–18.

Paredes, A.; Hood, W. R.; Seymour, H.; and Gollob, M. 1973. "Loss of Control in Alcoholism: An Investigation of the Hypothesis with Experimental Findings." *Quarterly Journal of Studies on Alcohol* 34:1146–61.

Partanen, J.; Bruun, K.; and Markham, T. 1966. *Inheritance of Drinking Behavior*. New Brunswick, N.J.: Rutgers University Center of Alcohol Studies.

Pattison, E. Mansell. 1966. "A Critique of Alcoholism Treatment Concepts with Special Reference to Abstinence." *Quarterly Journal of Studies on Alcohol* 27:49–71.

———. 1977. "Ten Years of Change in Alcoholism Treatment Findings." *American Journal of Psychiatry* 134:261–66.

———. 1985. "The Selection of Treatment Modalities for the Alcoholic Patient." In Mendelson and Mello (1985), 189–294.

Pattison, E. Mansell; Sobell, Mark B.; and Sobell, Linda C. 1977. *Emerging Concepts of Alcohol Dependence.* New York: Springer.

Peele, Stanton. 1984. "The Cultural Context of Psychological Approaches to Alcoholism." *American Psychologist* 39, no. 12.

———. 1985. *The Meaning of Addiction.* Lexington, Mass.: D. C. Heath.

———. 1986. Unpublished letter to SPSSI Study of Threats to Academic Freedom.

———. 1987a. "The Limitations of Control-of-Supply Models for Explaining and Preventing Alcoholism and Drug Addiction." *Journal of Studies on Alcoholism* 48:61–77.

———. 1987b. "What Does Addiction Have to Do with Level of Consumption? A Response to R. Room." *Journal of Alcohol Studies* 48:84–89.

———, ed. 1987c. *Visions of Addiction. Journal of Drug Issues* 17, nos. 1 and 2 [special issue].

Pendery, Mary L.; Maltzman, Irving M.; and West, L. Jolyon. 1982. "Controlled Drinking by Alcoholics? New Findings and a Reevaluation of a Major Affirmative Study." *Science* 217:169–75.

Pittman, David J. 1983. "An Evaluation of the Control of Consumption Policy." In Grant (1983), 159–72.

Polich, J. Michael. 1980. "Patterns of Remission in Alcoholism." In Edwards and Grant (1980), 95–112.

Polich, J. Michael; Armor, David J.; and Braiker, Harriet B. 1980. *The Course of Alcoholism: Four Years After Treatment.* Santa Monica, Calif.: The Rand Corporation.

Polich, J. Michael, and Kaelber, Charles T. 1985. "Sample Surveys and the Epidemiology of Alcoholism." In Schuckit (1985c), 43–77.

Pomerleau, O.; Pertschuk, M.; and Stinnent, J. 1976. "A Critical Examination of Some Current Assumptions in the Treatment of Alcoholism." *Journal of Studies on Alcohol* 37:849–67.

Popham, R. E., and Schmidt, W. 1976. "Some Factors Affecting the Likelihood of Moderate Drinking by Treated Alcoholics." *Journal of Studies on Alcohol* 37:868–82.

Popham, R. E.; Schmidt, W.; and Israelstam, Stephen. 1985. "Heavy

Alcohol Consumption and Physical Health Problems." In Schuckit (1985c), 203–46.

Reinert, R. E. 1968. "The Concept of Alcoholism as a Disease." *Bulletin of the Menninger Clinic* 32:21–25.

Robinson, David. 1976. "Factors Influencing Alcohol Consumption." In Edwards and Grant (1976): 60–77.

———. 1979. *Talking Out of Alcoholism*. London: Croom Helm.

Rodin, Miriam B. 1981. "Alcoholism as a Folk Disease." *Journal of Studies on Alcohol* 42:822–35.

Rohan, William P. 1978. "Comments on the NCA Criteria Study." *Journal of Studies on Alcohol* 39:211–18.

Roizen, Ron. 1987. "The Great Controlled-Drinking Controversy." In M. Galanter, ed., *Recent Developments in Alcoholism*, 5:245–79. New York: Plenum Press.

Room, Robin. 1977. "Measurement and Distribution of Drinking Patterns and Problems in General Populations." In Edwards et al. (1977), 61–88.

———. 1978. *Governing Images of Alcohol and Drug Problems: The Structure, Sources, and Sequels of Conceptualizations of Intractable Problems*. Berkeley, Calif.: Social Research Group.

———. 1980. "Treatment-Seeking Populations and Larger Realities." In Edwards and Grant (1980), 205–24.

———. 1983. "Sociological Aspects of the Disease Concept of Alcoholism." In Smart et al. (1983), 47–92.

———. 1987. "Alcohol Control, Addiction, and Processes of Change: A Comment on 'The Limitations of Control-of-Supply Models for Explaining and Preventing Alcoholism and Drug Addiction.'" *Journal of Alcohol Studies* 48:78–83.

Room, Robin, and Collins, Gary, eds. 1981. *Alcohol and Disinhibition: Nature and Meaning of the Link*. Rockville, Md.: Department of Health and Human Services, National Institute on Alcohol Abuse and Alcoholism.

Rorabaugh, W. J. 1979. *The Alcoholic Republic*. Oxford: Oxford University Press.

Royce, James E. 1981. *Alcohol Problems and Alcoholism*. New York: Free Press.

Rudy, David R. 1986. *Becoming Alcoholic*. Carbondale: Southern Illinois University Press.

Rush, Brian R., and Ogborne, Alan C. 1986. "Acceptability of Nonabstinence Treatment Goals Among Alcoholism Treatment Programs." *Journal of Studies on Alcohol* 47:146–49.

Saxe, Leonard; Dougherty, Denise; Esty, Katherine; and Fine, Michelle. 1983. "The Effectiveness and Costs of Alcoholism Treatment." Health Technology Case Study 22. Washington, D.C.: Office of Technology Assessment.

Saxe, Leonard; Dougherty, Denise; Esty, Katherine. 1985. "The Effectiveness and Cost of Alcoholism Treatment: A Public Policy Perspective." In Mendelson and Mello (1985), 485–539.

Schmidt, Wolfgang. 1976. "Cirrhosis and Alcohol Consumption: An Epidemiological Perspective." In Edwards and Grant (1976), 15–47.

Schuckit, Marc A. 1977. "Alcoholism: A Controlled Trial of 'Treatment' and 'Advice'" [comments]. *Journal of Studies on Alcohol* 38:1813–16.

———. 1980. "Charting What Has Changed." In Edwards and Grant (1980), 59–78.

———. 1984. *Drug and Alcohol Abuse.* New York: Plenum Press.

———. 1985a. "A One-Year Follow-up of Men Alcoholics Given Disulfiram." *Journal of Studies on Alcohol* 46:191–95.

———. 1985b. "Treatment of Alcoholism in Office and Outpatient Settings." In Mendelson and Mello (1985) 295–324.

———. 1985c. *Alcohol Patterns and Problems.* New Brunswick, N.J.: Rutgers University Press.

Schuckit, Marc A.; Goodwin, Donald A.; and Winokur, George. 1972. "A Study of Alcoholism in Half Siblings." *American Journal of Psychiatry* 128:123–27.

Schuckit, Marc A., and Viamontes, R. 1979. "Ethanol Ingestion: Differences in Blood Acetaldehyde Concentrations in Relatives of Alcoholics and Controls." *Science* 203:54.

Sells, S. B. 1981. "Matching Clients to Treatments: Problems, Preliminary Results, and Remaining Tasks." In Gottheil, McLellan, and Druley (1981), 33–50.

Shaw, Stan. 1985. "The Disease Concept of Dependence." In Heather, Robertson, and Davies (1985), 35–44.

Shaw, Stan; Cartwright, Alan; Spratley, Terry; and Harwin, Judith. 1978. *Responding to Drinking Problems.* London: Croom Helm.

Siegel, Shepard. 1983. "Classical Conditioning, Drug Tolerance and Drug Dependence." In Smart et al. (1983), 208–46.

Smart, Reginald G. 1975. "Spontaneous Recovery in Alcoholics: A Review and Analysis of the Available Research." *Drug and Alcohol Dependence* 1:277–85.

Smart, Reginald G.; Glaser, F. B.; Israel, Y.; Kalant, H.; Popham,

R. E.; and Schmidt, W., eds. 1983. *Research Advances in Alcohol and Drug Problems*, vol. 7. New York: Plenum Press.

Smart, Reginald G.; Cappell, H. D.; Glaser, F. B.; Israel, Y.; Kalant, H.; Popham, R.; Schmidt, W.; and Sellers, E. M., eds. 1984. *Research Advances in Alcohol and Drug Problems*, vol. 8. New York: Plenum Press.

Sobell, Linda C. 1982. "Behavioral Treatment of Out-patient Problem Drinkers [case no. 1]." In William M. Hay and Peter E. Nathan, eds., *Clinical Case Studies in the Behavioral Treatment of Alcoholism*, 73–103. New York: Plenum Press.

Sobell, Linda C., and Sobell, Mark B. 1982. "Alcohol Treatment Outcome Evaluation Methodology." In *Prevention, Intervention and Treatment: Concerns and Models*. Monograph no. 3, pp. 293–321. Washington, D.C.: Department of Health and Human Services, National Institute on Alcohol Abuse and Alcoholism.

Sobell, Mark B., and Sobell, Linda C. 1972. *Individualized Behavior Therapy for Alcoholics: Rationale, Procedures, Preliminary Results, and Appendix*. California Mental Health Research Monograph no. 13. California Department of Mental Hygiene.

———. 1978. *Behavioral Treatment of Alcohol Problems*. New York: Plenum Press.

———. 1984. "The Aftermath of Heresy: A Response to Pendery et al.'s (1982) Critique of 'Individualized Behavior Therapy for Alcoholics.'" *Behavioral Research Therapy* 22:413–40.

Stockwell, T. R.; Hodgson, R. J.; and Rankin, H. J. 1980. "The Experimental Production and Measurement of Craving for Alcohol." Unpublished manuscript. Addiction Research Center, Royal College of Psychiatry, London.

Sullivan, Cheryl. 1987. "New Device Takes Ignition Keys Out of the Hands of Drinking Drivers." *Christian Science Monitor*, July 20.

Tarter, Ralph E. 1978. "Etiology of Alcoholism: Interdisciplinary Integration." In Nathan, Marlatt, and Loberg (1978), 41–70.

Tennant, Forrest S., Jr. 1986. "Disulfiram Will Reduce Medical Complications but Not Cure Alcoholism." *JAMA, Journal of the American Medical Association* 256:1489.

Tuchfield, Barry S. 1981. "Spontaneous Remission in Alcoholics." *Journal of Studies on Alcohol* 42:626–41.

Tucker, Jalie A.; Vuchinich, Rudy E.; and Harris, Carole V. 1985. "Determinants of Substance Abuse Relapse." In Galizio and Maisto (1985), 383–421.

Vaillant, George E. 1980. "The Doctor's Dilemma." In Edwards and Grant (1980), 13–31.

————. 1983. *The Natural History of Alcoholism*. Cambridge, Mass.: Harvard University Press.

————. 1984. "The Contribution of Prospective Studies in the Understanding of Etiologic Factors in Alcoholism." In Smart et al. (1984), 265–89.

Vaillant, George E., and Milofsky, Eva S. 1982. "The Etiology of Alcoholism: A Prospective Viewpoint." *American Psychologist* 37: 494–503.

Viamontes, J. A. 1972. "Review of Drug Effectiveness in the Treatment of Alcoholism." *American Journal of Psychiatry* 128:1570–71.

Walsh, Brendan M. 1983. "The Economics of Alcohol Taxation." In Grant (1983), 173–89.

WHO Expert Committee on Problems Related to Alcohol Consumption. 1980. *Problems Related to Alcohol Consumption*. Technical Report Series 650. Geneva: World Health Organization.

Wiener, Carolyn L. 1981. *The Politics of Alcoholism*. New Brunswick, N.J.: Transaction Books.

Zucker, Robert A., and Gomberg, Edith L. 1986. "Etiology of Alcoholism Reconsidered: The Case for a Biopsychosocial Process." *American Psychologist* 41:783–93.

# INDEX

Abstinence, 13, 15, 19, 122; as treatment goal, 3, 4, 73, 121, 124
Acetaldehyde, 55
Addiction: other than alcoholism, 7
Alcohol: advertising, 138–39; amount drunk in U.S., 14, 16; availability to public, 137–39; as cause of drinking, 33–43; "Good Creature of God," 13, 16; as healthful, 14; regulation, 137–39; as socially valued, 14, 144
Alcoholic: varying meanings, 5, 49
Alcoholics: appropriate attitudes toward, 109–13; children of, 51–55, 61; and control over drinking, 34–41, 105, 110–11; definition unclear, 5; drinking patterns of, variation in, 21–22; expectations and beliefs, effect on drinking, 39; illness and death rates, 82, 126; motives, effect on drinking, 81, 108–9; with non-alcoholic parents, 51–53; number of in U.S., 5–6, 133; and problem drinkers, 4–6, 21, 137; as responsive to incentives and costs,

35–36, 37, 45; setting, effects on drinking, 36, 39–43, 64; as treatment counselors, 23–24. *See also* Alcoholism; Craving; Tolerance; Withdrawal
Alcoholics Anonymous (AA), 3; as advocates of disease concept, 18; doctrine and method, 20, 31, 87–88; evaluating efficacy, 88–90; origins, 18; self-selective membership, 89; as way of life, 90–91
Alcoholism, 6, 27; and anxiety, 58, 61, 86; "breakthroughs" in explaining, 27–28, 55; delta, 32–33; and dependency, 56–61; and depression, 58, 86; and family, 51; gamma, 20, 22, 33; genetic influence, 51–55, 62; health consequences, 74; and impulsivity, 61; and inner conflict, 61; and learning theories, 62–63; "maturing out" and spontaneous improvement, 21, 72, 77, 84, 92; and personality, 61; phases of, 3, 6, 19, 21; plurality of causes, 50; and